AF683443

DOCUMENTED BRIEFING

Effects of Preanalytical Variables on the Quality of Biospecimens Used to Study Genetic Changes in Cancer

Development of the Biospecimen Research Database

Elisa Eiseman

Sponsored by the National Cancer Institute

RAND Transportation, Space, and Technology

A RAND INFRASTRUCTURE, SAFETY, AND ENVIRONMENT PROGRAM

This research was sponsored by the National Cancer Institute and was conducted under the auspices of the Transportation, Space, and Technology (TST) Program within RAND Infrastructure, Safety, and Environment (ISE).

Published 2009 by the RAND Corporation
1776 Main Street, P.O. Box 2138, Santa Monica, CA 90407-2138
1200 South Hayes Street, Arlington, VA 22202-5050
4570 Fifth Avenue, Suite 600, Pittsburgh, PA 15213-2665
RAND URL: http://www.rand.org/
To order RAND documents or to obtain additional information, contact
Distribution Services: Telephone: (310) 451-7002;
Fax: (310) 451-6915; Email: order@rand.org

PREFACE

About This Document

The National Cancer Institute (NCI) Office of Biorepositories and Biospecimen Research (OBBR), established in 2005 to address the issues associated with the need for high-quality, well-annotated biospecimens for biomedical research, asked the RAND Corporation to identify and analyze existing data on the effects of preanalytical variables (i.e., environmental and biological variables introduced by acquisition, processing, storage, and distribution) on biospecimens used to study genetic and proteomic changes in cancer. The full implementation of this project was envisioned as a multiyear project consisting of three objectives: (1) to identify and analyze existing data on the effects of preanalytical variables on biospecimens used to study genetic and proteomic changes in cancer; (2) to create an interactive, searchable Web site that scientists, pathologists, repositories, and others can visit to learn about and contribute data, methods, and other relevant information on how biospecimens used to study genetic and proteomic changes in cancer are affected by preanalytical variables; and (3) to provide information to the research community and other interested parties about the effects of preanalytical variables on the quality of biospecimens used to study genetic and proteomic changes in cancer. The project was broken down into three phases. This documented briefing, which focuses on work conducted during the first year of this project, describes the process used to identify and analyze data on the effects of preanalytical variables on biospecimens used to study genetic and proteomic changes in cancer. It provides details on the development of the Biospecimen Research Database, a data-curation tool developed to provide a standardized way of consistently recording data on the effects of preanalytical variables, and summarizes the findings of the first phase of the study.

This documented briefing is based on the briefing given to OBBR on September 27, 2007, and is the final reporting requirement of the subcontract between BioReliance, Invitrogen Bioservices, and the RAND Corporation in support of the prime contract with NCI . This document provides OBBR with a framework for analyzing the effects of preanalytical variables on various biospecimen types, research questions, and analytic methods. This document should also be of interest to investigators, pathologists, and biorepositories that collect, store, distribute, or use biospecimens for research purposes. The ultimate goal of the database is to provide information to OBBR and the scientific community that will optimize the quality, accessibility, and utility of biospecimens for research purposes.

The RAND Transportation, Space, and Technology Program

This research was conducted under the auspices of the Transportation, Space, and Technology (TST) Program within RAND Infrastructure, Safety, and Environment (ISE). The mission of RAND Infrastructure, Safety, and Environment is to improve the development, operation, use, and protection of society's essential physical assets and natural resources and to enhance the related social assets of safety and security of individuals in transit and in their workplaces and communities. The TST research portfolio encompasses policy areas including transportation systems, space exploration, information and telecommunication technologies, nano- and biotechnologies, and other aspects of science and technology policy.

Questions or comments about this briefing should be sent to the project leader, Elisa Eiseman (Elisa_Eiseman@rand.org). Information about the Transportation, Space, and Technology Program is available online (http://www.rand.org/ise/tech). Inquiries about TST research should be sent to the following address:

Martin Wachs, Director
Transportation, Space, and Technology Program, ISE
RAND Corporation
1776 Main Street
P. O. Box 2138
Santa Monica, CA 90401-2138
310-393-0411, x7720
Martin_Wachs@rand.org

CONTENTS

FIGURES

SUMMARY

Human biospecimens[1] are valuable research tools because they reflect the state of the biospecimen at the time it was collected. That is, the expression pattern of genes and proteins depends on both the biological state of the biospecimen (e.g., whether it is lung or colon tissue; whether it is diseased or normal) and the environmental and biological stresses the biospecimen experiences prior to analysis (i.e., preanalytical variables). Examples of preanalytical variables include

- medical or surgical procedures conducted before and during the removal of the biospecimen from the patient (e.g., administration of antibiotics, anesthesia, and other drugs; disruption of blood supply to the tissue; or intraoperative administration of blood, blood products or other fluids)
- biospecimen-processing methods (e.g., type of fixative, time in fixative, method and rate of freezing)
- duration and conditions of biospecimen transport and storage (e.g., storage and transport temperature, duration of storage).

Molecular analyses of biospecimens from cancers and other diseases have revealed changes in gene and protein expression (e.g., either over- or underexpression of specific genes). It is interesting to note that many of the same genes reported to have altered expression in diseases have also been shown to change expression in response to environmental changes and biological stresses. For example, it is clear from studies on yeast, plants, and animals that changes in temperature, pH, and nutrient availability; oxygen deprivation; and other environmental stresses can cause major changes in gene expression (Storey and Storey, 2001; Steinberg, Stürzenbaum, and Menzel, 2008; Kenneth and Rocha, 2008; Van Elzen, Moens, and Dewilde, 2008). Significant changes in gene expression can occur as early as 15 minutes after exposure to a stimulus or stress, while posttranslational changes in proteins, such as methylation and

---

[1] Human biospecimens include everything from subcellular structures (e.g., DNA, mRNA, proteins) to cells, tissue (bone, muscle, connective tissue, and skin), organs (e.g., liver, bladder, heart, kidney), blood, gametes (sperm and ova), embryos, fetal tissue, and waste (urine, feces, sweat, hair and nail clippings, shed epithelial cells, placenta).

phosphorylation, can occur within seconds (Eastmond and Nelson, 2006; Kawasaki et al., 2001; Eiseman and Bolen, 1992). Since the value of a biospecimen to a researcher is the information it contains about the actual biological state of the specimen as it existed in the person from whom it was derived, determining which changes are disease-related and which are artifacts caused by preanalytical variables is of utmost importance.

The scientific community has repeatedly identified the limited availability of carefully collected and controlled, high-quality human biospecimens annotated with essential clinical data and properly consented for broad investigational use as the leading obstacle to progress in postgenomics cancer research (OBBR, undated [c]). The National Cancer Institute (NCI) is leading a national initiative to systematically address and resolve this problem. Since 2002, when NCI leadership identified biorepositories as an area of critical importance, NCI has been involved in several efforts to determine best practices for biospecimen collection and management. In support of this effort, NCI established the Office of Biorepositories and Biospecimen Research (OBBR) in 2005 to address the issues associated with the need for high-quality, well-annotated biospecimens for biomedical research.

OBBR's mission is "to ensure that human specimens available for cancer research are of the highest quality" (OBBR, undated [a]). To accomplish its mission, OBBR has established biobanking as a new area of research and conducts and funds research on the effects of preanalytical variables on the usefulness of biospecimens in genomic and proteomic studies (OBBR, undated [c]). The results of the research sponsored by OBBR will support the development of guidelines and evidence-based standards for biospecimens and biorepositories that will optimize the quality and accessibility of biospecimens for the cancer and broader biomedical research communities.

One of the questions in which OBBR was interested was what, if any, data exist on the effects of preanalytical variables on biospecimens. To begin to answer this question, OBBR asked RAND to identify and analyze existing data on the effects of these variables on biospecimens used to study genetic and proteomic changes in cancer. The full implementation of this project was envisioned as a multiyear project consisting of three objectives: (1) to identify and analyze existing data on the effects of preanalytical variable on biospecimens used to study genetic and proteomic changes in cancer; (2) to create an interactive, searchable Web site that scientists, pathologists, repositories, and others can visit to learn about and contribute data, methods, and other relevant information on how biospecimens used to study genetic and proteomic changes in cancer are affected by preanalytical variables; and (3) to provide information to the research community and other interested parties about the effects of preanalytical variables on the quality of biospecimens used to study genetic and proteomic changes in cancer. The information generated by this project was intended to provide OBBR with insight into the molecular impacts of different preanalytical variables on different biospecimen types, research questions, and analysis methods.

This documented briefing, which focuses on work conducted during the first year of this multiphase project, describes the process used to identify and analyze data on the effects of preanalytical variables on biospecimens used to study genetic and proteomic changes in cancer. It provides details on the development of the Biospecimen Research Database, a data-curation tool developed to provide a standardized way of consistently recording data on the effects of preanalytical variables, and summarizes the findings of the first phase of the study.

Developing the Data-Curation Tool

To make the findings of this project useful to the scientific community, it was necessary to develop a systematic way of capturing the wealth of data collected through the review of the scientific literature. A data-curation tool, called the Biospecimen Research Database, was developed to provide a standardized way of consistently recording data obtained through the literature review. Developing the data-curation tool involved several activities. First, the major subject-area headings and specific fields for data collection had to be defined. Next, a data-accession tool needed to be designed. A preliminary template was designed using a Microsoft Excel spreadsheet, which was pilot tested to determine whether the appropriate data-collection fields had been selected. A more user-friendly, interactive data-accession tool was then designed using a Microsoft Access database, which was also pilot tested to assess its usability and robustness.

The first step in developing the data-curation tool was to determine the types of data that would be collected from the literature review. The types of data to be collected were grouped into six major subject areas of interest: biospecimen type, tissue type, diagnosis, biomolecule type, technology platform, and experimental factors. Next, specific fields for data collection within each major subject-area heading were identified. The major subject-area headings and associated specific data-entry fields went through several revisions during the development of the Excel and Access data-curation tools.

A preliminary data-collection template was developed using an Excel spreadsheet. The Excel data-collection template was pilot tested to assess its usability and robustness. The template was refined by the addition and deletion of data-entry fields based on the type and importance of information found during the pilot test.

The Access database curation tool was developed in collaboration with OBBR. The fields defined in the Excel data-collection template formed the basis of the Access database curation tool. Data-entry forms with drop-down menus and free-text boxes were developed to improve the ease of data entry. Two different forms were developed: one to capture general information about the paper and one to capture specific data about the studies within the paper. The Access database curation tool was pilot tested to provide a direct comparison to the Excel template, confirm its usability and robustness, and provide indications of where revisions of data-entry fields were necessary.

The Access database curation tool formed the basis for the development of an online data-collection Web site. The online data-collection Web site, which is still under development, was designed in such a way that, as data are entered, they directly populate an online, searchable database. The data-collection Web site and the searchable Biospecimen Research Database, which contains data on the effects of preanalytical variables on the quality of biospecimens, is being built by OBBR with input from RAND and hosted on the OBBR external Web site. A prototype version is available online as a Web-based, searchable database that provides information about the effects of preanalytical variables on biospecimens (see OBBR, undated [d]).

Literature-Search Strategies

A comprehensive search of the scientific literature was performed to identify studies conducted specifically to determine the effects of preanalytical variables on the quality of biospecimens used to study genetic and proteomic changes in cancer. To accomplish this, RAND developed a literature-search strategy designed to find studies of interest. Papers were selected to populate the database using several literature-search strategies, including keyword searches, MeSH® term searches, and author searches.

Keyword and MeSH term searches of PubMed were conducted using a targeted set of search terms to find relevant articles. Searches ranged from very specific (such as the keyword search for *preanalytical variable* and variations thereof and the MeSH term search for *tissue fixation*) to very broad, general searches (such as those using variations of the terms *human*, *specimen*, *acquisition*, *processing*, *storage*, *effect*, *gene*, *protein*, *DNA*, *RNA*, and *analysis*). Other relevant Web sites were also searched, including journals that feature biological methods (e.g., *BioTechniques*, *Cell Preservation Technology* [now *Biopreservation and Biobanking*]). Searches for relevant studies also included the examination of the reference lists of articles already retrieved. In addition, a search of PubMed was performed to identify relevant papers authored by a target list of investigators who are active in the field of biospecimen research. Of all the searches, the search using the MeSH term *tissue fixation* yielded the highest percentage of relevant papers. Virtually all of the papers identified by this search were relevant, and almost 30 percent of the papers were analyzed and included in the database.

The time period specified for the searches covered the past 20 years (i.e., from 1987 through 2007). While many relevant studies were found in papers published more than 10 years ago (i.e., papers published before 1997), it was decided that more recent papers (i.e., papers published between 1997 and 2007) would be of most relevance to the research community and were selected as a place to start to populate the database. Search results were also limited to English-language publications. Only studies that used human biospecimens were included in the database; studies using biospecimens from other animal sources were not analyzed. Also, only original research articles were included in the database; review articles were not included.

Data Analysis and Study Results

The effects of preanalytical variables on the molecular profile of biospecimens will differ depending on the specimen type (e.g., blood, urine, normal tissue, cancerous tissue), the biomolecule being analyzed (e.g., DNA, RNA, protein), the analysis method being used (e.g., Southern blot, polymerase chain reaction [PCR], fluorescent in situ hybridization [FISH], cDNA microarrays), and the research question being asked. One way to conceptualize these preanalytical variables and their potential effects is to array them according to the biospecimen type, the analysis method, and the research question being asked (Figure S.1) (Barker et al., 2005). The three-dimensional array has the biospecimen types along the x-axis, the biomolecule types and associated analysis methods along the y-axis, and the research questions along the z-axis (the blue, red, and off-white colors depict different research questions). This array, developed by OBBR, provides a useful framework for the analysis of the effects of preanalytical variables on biospecimens. By systematically filling in the boxes in the array for each biospecimen type with information about the effects of preanalytical variables on the technology platform used and the research question asked, insight can be gained into the specific impact of different preanalytical variables on the molecular profile of the biospecimen.

At the time of the briefing to OBBR, 145 studies from 65 papers had been analyzed and entered into the database. The number of studies per paper ranged from one to eight, with most papers containing two to three studies. Of the 145 studies, 45 studies analyzed DNA as the biomolecule,

Figure S.1. Framework for Analysis of Effects of Preanalytical Variables on Biospecimens

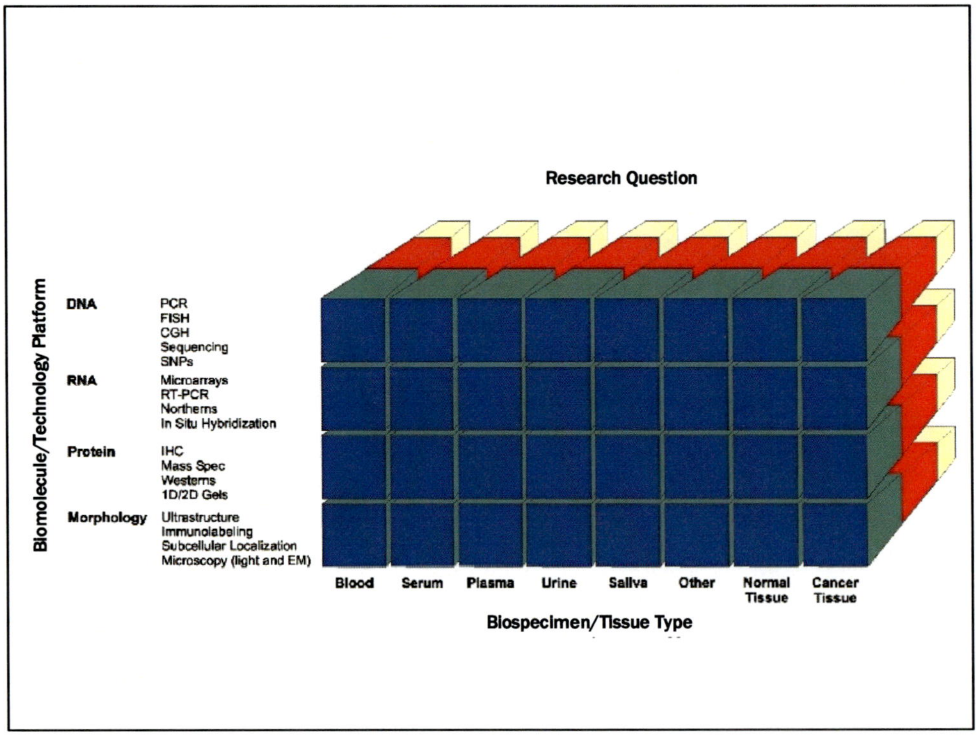

46 analyzed RNA, 53 analyzed proteins, and 10 analyzed morphology[2] (note that each study may include more than one biomolecule type). Currently, there are data from 193 studies from 80 papers in the database.

The studies used 22 different technology platforms and reported on 15 preanalytical variables. The most commonly used technology platforms were reverse transcription PCR (RT-PCR) to analyze RNA, immunohistochemistry to analyze proteins, and PCR to analyze DNA. The most commonly investigated preanalytical variables were type of fixative, biomolecule extraction method, time at room temperature/pre-fixation time, and time in fixative. Most preanalytical variables had several associated values. The number of associated values ranged from one to eight, with most preanalytical variables having two associated values. For example, *time in fixative* typically had several associated values, since each time point in an experiment using a time course would be a new value (e.g., 15 minutes, 30 minutes, 1 hour, 2 hours, 3 hours, 4 hours, 5 hours).

Challenges and Next Steps

There are some challenges when it comes to analyzing the data in the Biospecimen Research Database. Data on the effects of preanalytical variables on biospecimens are not reported consistently in the literature, a fact that may make comparisons between studies and analyses across studies difficult (i.e., meta-analysis). For example, one study may report time in weeks (e.g., 4 weeks), while another may report it in months (e.g., 0 to 1 month). It is important to determine whether these different measures of time are comparable when performing meta-analyses. The database may be most useful as a tool to identify gaps in research on the effects of preanalytical variables on biospecimens in which additional studies may be valuable.

Consistency in recording data in the database is also crucial to be able to make comparisons between studies and perform meta-analyses. Drop-down menus with controlled vocabularies were used to help prevent

---

[2] *Morphology* is the study of the size, shape, and structure of a particular organism, organ, tissue, or cell. For the purposes of this briefing, the term *morphology* refers to the examination of the detailed structure of cells and tissues (sometimes called *cellular morphology*). Techniques used to study the morphology of cells and tissues include histology, immunohistochemistry, in situ hybridization, electron microscopy, and light, fluorescent, and confocal microscopy.

variation from being introduced into the database by the curation process. Limiting or even eliminating the use of free-text boxes to record important findings would also be helpful. Another way in which variation was controlled was by using a second reviewer to check the accuracy of the entries in the database and ensure consistency across data entered by different curators.

Another challenge in analyzing the data is the way in which the effects of preanalytical variables (i.e., the results of the studies) are recorded. Currently, preanalytical variables are selected from a drop-down menu in the data-curation tool, allowing researchers using the Biospecimen Research Database to easily identify which preanalytical variables were investigated in the study. In contrast, the results of the study are recorded in a free-text box (i.e., "Summary of Findings"), making it more difficult to identify what effect, if any, the preanalytical variable had on the biospecimen used, the biomolecule analyzed, or the research question asked. A more systematic way is needed to record and easily identify which preanalytical variables had an effect and what those effects were.

The next steps for the Biospecimen Research Database include expanding the information in the database with data from additional studies that focus directly on the effects of preanalytical variables on biospecimens, as well as adding information from clinical laboratory testing procedures relevant to research on genetic and proteomic changes in cancer (e.g., genetic testing, cytogenetics, molecular pathology). Information may also be obtained from studies that address preanalytical effects as part of the methodology section of the paper. In addition, information may be available from technical-support documents that accompany products used to collect, process, store, transport, or analyze biospecimens (e.g., DNA and RNA purification kits, DNA sequencers, real-time PCR machines). Eventually, it may be feasible to obtain unpublished data on the effects of preanalytical variables on biospecimens from investigators who are active in the field of biospecimen research.

As the database grows, it will be possible to fill in more boxes in the array and to fill each box with sufficient information to be able to start performing analyses of the effects of preanalytical variables on the biospecimens. These data could be used to identify gaps in knowledge about the effects of preanalytical variables and to support the development of guidelines and evidence-based standards for the collection, processing, and storage of biospecimens. The ultimate goal of the database is to provide information to OBBR and the scientific community that will optimize the quality, accessibility, and utility of biospecimens for research purposes.

ACKNOWLEDGMENTS

The author wishes to thank the staff from the National Cancer Institute (NCI) Office of Biorepositories and Biospecimen Research, Helen Moore, Ph.D., Biospecimen Research Network Program Manager, and Jim Vaught, Ph.D., Deputy Director, for their guidance and support in carrying out this work. The author also wishes to thank Ian Fore, D. Phil., Director, Biospecimen and Pathology Informatics, NCI Center for Bioinformatics, for his technical expertise with bioinformatics systems. The author wishes to thank Asha Pathak, John A. Zambrano, and Anant Patel, who contributed by helping with the development of the data-curation tools and reviewing papers that are included in the Biospecimen Research Database. The author also wishes to thank the reviewers for this documented briefing, Stuart S. Olmsted, Ph.D. Natural Scientist, RAND Corporation, and Waqas Amin, M.D., Postdoctoral Fellow in Biomedical Informatics, University of Pittsburgh, for their insightful and timely reviews. The author also wishes to thank Lisa Bernard, who edited this documented briefing.

ABBREVIATIONS

1D	one dimensional
2D	two dimensional
CGH	comparative genomic hybridization
cDNA	complementary deoxyribonucleic acid
DNA	deoxyribonucleic acid
CSF	cerebrospinal fluid
ELISA	enzyme-linked immunosorbant assay
EM	electron microscopy
FISH	fluorescent in situ hybridization
H&E	hematoxylin and eosin
IHC	immunohistochemistry
ISE	RAND Infrastructure, Safety, and Environment
LC-MS	liquid chromatography–mass spectrometry
MALDI	matrix-assisted laser desorption/ionization
NBN	National Biospecimen Network
NCI	National Cancer Institute
OBBR	Office of Biorepositories and Biospecimen Research
OCT	optimum cutting temperature (an embedding compound used in freezing specimens)
PCR	polymerase chain reaction
PSA	prostate-specific antigen
PTH	parathyroid hormone
RNA	ribonucleic acid

RT-PCR	reverse transcription polymerase chain reaction
SELDI	surface-enhanced laser desorption/ionization
SNP	single nucleotide polymorphism
SOP	standard operating procedure
TOF	time-of-flight
TST	Transportation, Space, and Technology

CHAPTER ONE. INTRODUCTION

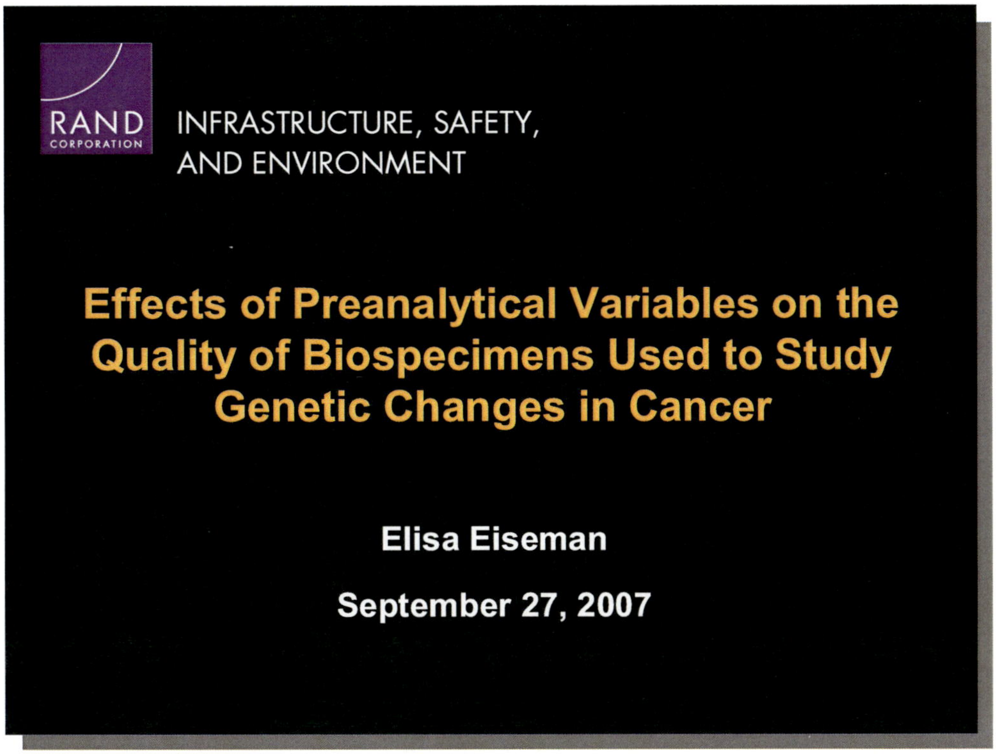

Human biospecimens[1] and associated demographic and clinical data are collected and stored for research purposes at hundreds of biorepositories throughout the United States.[2] Researchers use these valuable biospecimens to study the molecular characteristics of disease by providing information about the physiologic or pathologic condition of the person from whom they are derived. Sequencing of the human genome, advances in genomic and proteomic research, and a focus on

---

[1] Human biospecimens include everything from subcellular structures (e.g., DNA, mRNA, proteins) to cells, tissue (bone, muscle, connective tissue, and skin), organs (e.g., liver, bladder, heart, kidney), blood, gametes (sperm and ova), embryos, fetal tissue, and waste (urine, feces, sweat, hair and nail clippings, shed epithelial cells, placenta).

[2] A 1999 RAND study conservatively estimated that there were more than 307 million human biospecimens from more than 178 million cases stored in the United States, accumulating at a rate of more than 20 million specimens per year (Eiseman and Haga, 1999).

pharmacogenomics have placed a renewed emphasis on the need for high-quality, well-annotated biospecimens, collected with robust informed consent to advance our understanding of the genetic basis of such diseases as cancer, HIV/AIDS, and heart disease.

While it seems that there should be plenty of biospecimens available for research use, there are several complicating factors. One of the major impediments is that biospecimens are collected, processed, stored, and distributed differently from one biorepository to the next, which introduces variability and complicates comparisons of research results obtained using biospecimens from different biorepositories. These differences occur primarily because there is no standardization or harmonization between biorepositories. Every repository that exists today was established to fulfill a specific set of objectives, and the design and operations of each repository is integrally linked to those objectives (Eiseman, Bloom, et al., 2003). Therefore, techniques for biospecimen collection, processing, storage, and distribution—the core functions of a biorepository—vary depending on the purpose for which the repository was established. Likewise, the quality and extent of information collected with the specimens vary depending on the purpose for which the specimen was originally collected. The type of informed consent— general surgical consent versus specific informed consent for the use of the biospecimen for research purposes—also varies from repository to repository, sometimes limiting the usefulness of some biospecimens for certain kinds of research. Therefore, biospecimens currently stored at biorepositories may be of limited use for certain types of genomics- and proteomics-based research due to the method in which they were collected, processed, or stored (e.g., paraffin embedded instead of snap frozen), a lack of sufficient clinical data, or the type of informed consent. In addition, the lack of nationally agreed-on quality control and standard operating procedures (SOPs) for the collection, processing, storage, and distribution of biospecimens limits the usefulness of existing collections for research requiring highly standardized specimen collection and preparation.

The scientific community has repeatedly identified limited availability of carefully collected and controlled, high-quality human biospecimens annotated with essential clinical data and properly consented for broad investigational use as the leading obstacle to progress in postgenomics cancer research (OBBR, undated [c]). The National Cancer Institute (NCI) is leading a national initiative to systematically address and resolve this problem. Since 2002, when NCI leadership identified biorepositories as an area of critical importance, NCI has been involved in several efforts to determine best practices for biospecimen collection and management, including seeking input from leaders in the fields of cancer research, clinical oncology, pathology, patient advocacy and private industry; commissioning a report from the RAND Corporation on biorepository best practices (Eiseman, Bloom, et al., 2003); collaborating on the National Biospecimen Network (NBN) Blueprint; conducting an internal study of NCI-funded biorepositories; establishing the Biorepository Coordinating Committee; convening two national workshops ("Best Practices for Biorepositories That Support Cancer Research" and "Biospecimen Ethical, Legal, and Policy Issues"); and establishing the Office of Biorepositories and Biospecimen Research (OBBR) (OBBR, undated [b]).

OBBR was established by NCI in 2005 to address the issues associated with the need for high-quality, well-annotated biospecimens for biomedical research. Its mission is "to ensure that human specimens available for cancer research are of the highest quality" (OBBR, undated [a]). To accomplish its mission, OBBR has established biobanking as a new area of research and conducts and funds research on the effects of various collection and processing protocols (preanalytical variables[3]) on the usefulness of biospecimens in genomic and proteomic studies (OBBR, undated [c]). The results of the research sponsored by OBBR will support the development of guidelines and evidence-based standards for biospecimens and biorepositories that will optimize the quality and accessibility of biospecimens for the cancer and broader biomedical research communities. However, before OBBR committed funds to this area of research, it wanted to know what, if any, data exist on the effects of preanalytical variables on biospecimens. To begin to answer this question, OBBR asked RAND to identify and analyze any existing data on the effects of these variables on biospecimens used to study genetic and proteomic changes in cancer. Specifically, OBBR has requested that RAND focus on data on the effects of preanalytical variables on the research questions, biospecimen types, and analysis methods to be studied by OBBR in the establishment of its Biospecimen Research Network.

The information generated by this project will provide OBBR with insight into the molecular impacts of different preanalytical variables on different

---

[3] *Preanalytical variables* are circumstances occurring before specimen collection, specimen collection itself, and handling of the specimen prior to analysis. Examples of preanalytical variables include normal physiological responses (e.g., a patient's response to anesthesia) and specimen-collection factors (e.g., time of sampling, materials and methods used for sampling, and duration and conditions of sample transport and storage before the measurements—e.g., freezing and thawing of serum).

biospecimen types, research questions, and analysis methods. This documented briefing describes the process used to identify and analyze data on the effects of preanalytical variables on biospecimens used to study genetic and proteomic changes in cancer. It provides details on the development of the Biospecimen Research Database, which contains information about the effects of preanalytical variables, and summarizes the findings of the study.

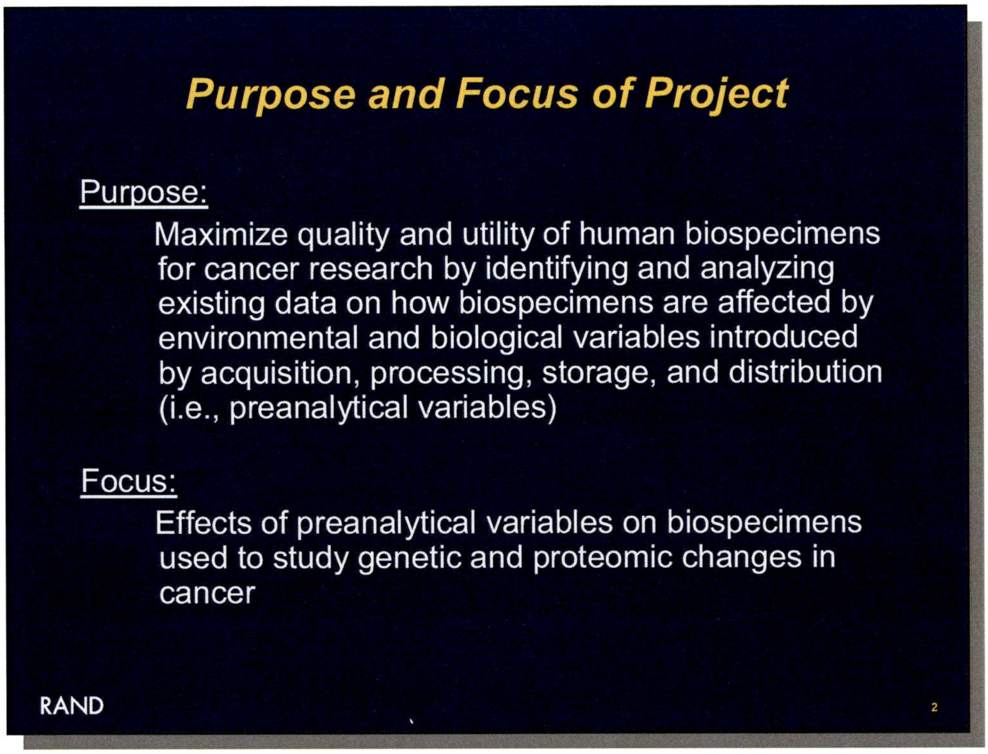

Before biological material is removed from a person and becomes a biospecimen, it first exists in situ within a specific biologic context, which is reflected in its molecular profile (i.e., the pattern of expression of genes and proteins). At any point during the acquisition, processing, storage, and distribution of a biospecimen, environmental and biological variables may be introduced that can alter the molecular profile of the specimen. Examples of events that may affect the molecular profile of a biospecimen include the following:

- acquisition: medical or surgical procedures conducted during the removal of the biospecimen from the patient (e.g., administration of antibiotics, anesthesia, and other drugs; disruption of blood supply to the tissue [warm ischemic time]; intraoperative administration of blood, blood products, or other fluids; handling of the specimen in the operating room; transport and delivery to the pathologist; and isolation of the biospecimen by the pathologist)
- processing: procedures used during isolation, purification, fixation, and preservation of the biospecimen (e.g., time at room temperature, temperature of room, type of fixative, time in fixative, method and rate of freezing, and size of specimen aliquots)
- storage: storage temperature, duration of storage, and progressive dehydration, desiccation, or oxidation

- distribution: transport conditions (e.g., shipped in liquid nitrogen, on dry ice, or at ambient temperature).

Once it is removed from a person, a biospecimen reflects the state of the specimen at the time it was collected—i.e., the expression pattern of genes and proteins will depend on both the biological state of the biospecimen (e.g., whether it is lung or colon tissue; whether it is diseased or normal) and the environmental and biological stresses the biospecimen experiences during the processes of acquisition, processing, storage, and distribution (i.e., preanalytical variables). Since the value of a biospecimen to a researcher is the information it contains about the actual biological state of the specimen as it existed in the person from whom it was derived, determining which changes are disease-related and which are artifacts is of utmost importance.

Furthermore, molecular analyses of biospecimens from people with cancer or other diseases often reveal changes in gene and protein expression (e.g., either over- or underexpression of specific genes). However, many of the same genes reported to have altered expression in diseases have also been shown to change expression in response to environmental modifications and biological stresses. For example, it is clear from studies on yeast, plants, and animals that changes in temperature, pH, and nutrient availability; oxygen deprivation; and other environmental stresses can cause major changes in gene expression (Storey and Storey, 2001; Steinberg, Stürzenbaum, and Menzel, 2008; Kenneth and Rocha, 2008; van Elzen, Moens, and Dewilde, 2008). Significant changes in gene expression can occur as early as 15 minutes after exposure to a stimulus or stress, while posttranslational changes in proteins, such as methylation and phosphorylation, can occur within seconds (Eastmond and Nelson, 2006; Kawasaki et al., 2001; Eiseman and Bolen, 1992). Therefore, determining which changes are disease-related and which may have been introduced by environmental changes and biological stresses that occur during the acquisition, processing, storage, and distribution of the biospecimen is not trivial.

The purpose of this project was to maximize the quality and utility of human biospecimens for cancer research by identifying and analyzing existing data on how biospecimens are affected by environmental and biological variables introduced by acquisition, processing, storage, and distribution (i.e., preanalytical variables). Specifically, this project focused on the effects of preanalytical variables on biospecimens used to study genetic and proteomic changes in cancer.

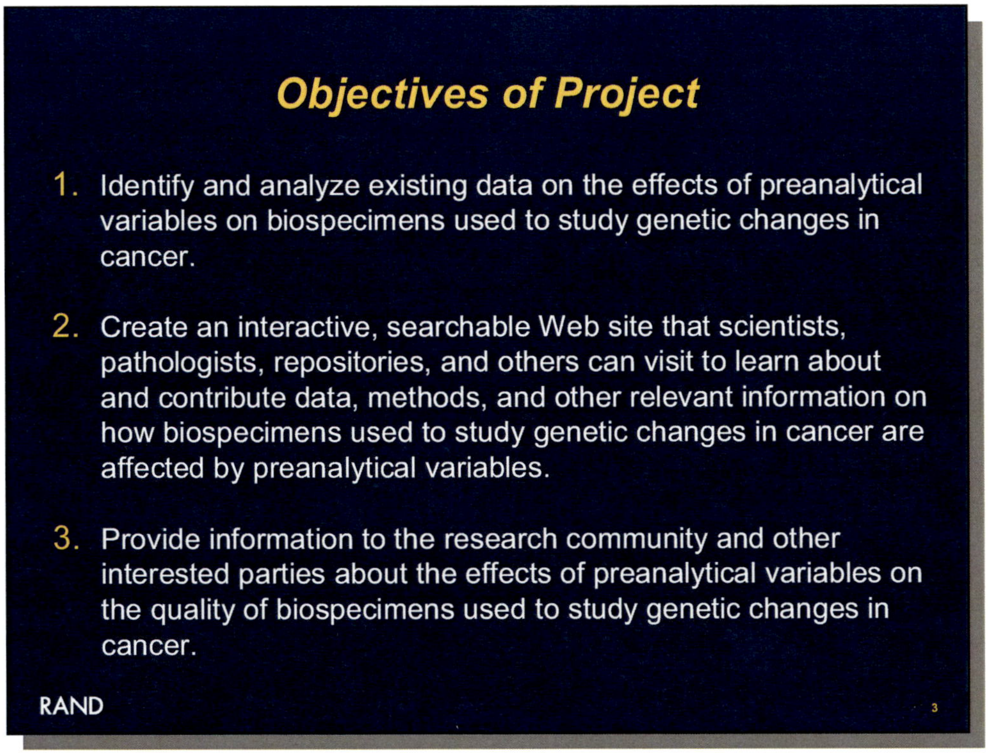

The objectives of this project are to do the following:

1. Identify and analyze existing data on the effects of preanalytical variables on biospecimens used to study genetic and proteomic changes in cancer by
    - conducting a comprehensive search of the scientific literature
    - reviewing clinical laboratory testing procedures relevant to research on genetic and proteomic changes in cancer (e.g., genetic testing, cytogenetics, molecular pathology)
    - examining information about products used to collect, process, store, transport, and analyze biospecimens (e.g., DNA and RNA purification kits, DNA sequencers, real-time polymerase chain reaction [PCR] machines) for information on the effects of preanalytical variables on biospecimens
    - requesting information from the scientific community about the effects of preanalytical variables on biospecimens
2. Create an interactive, searchable Web site that scientists, pathologists, repositories, and others can visit to learn about and contribute data, methods, and other relevant information on how biospecimens used to

study genetic and proteomic changes in cancer are affected by preanalytical variables.

3. Provide information to the research community and other interested parties about the effects of preanalytical variables on the quality of biospecimens used to study genetic and proteomic changes in cancer.

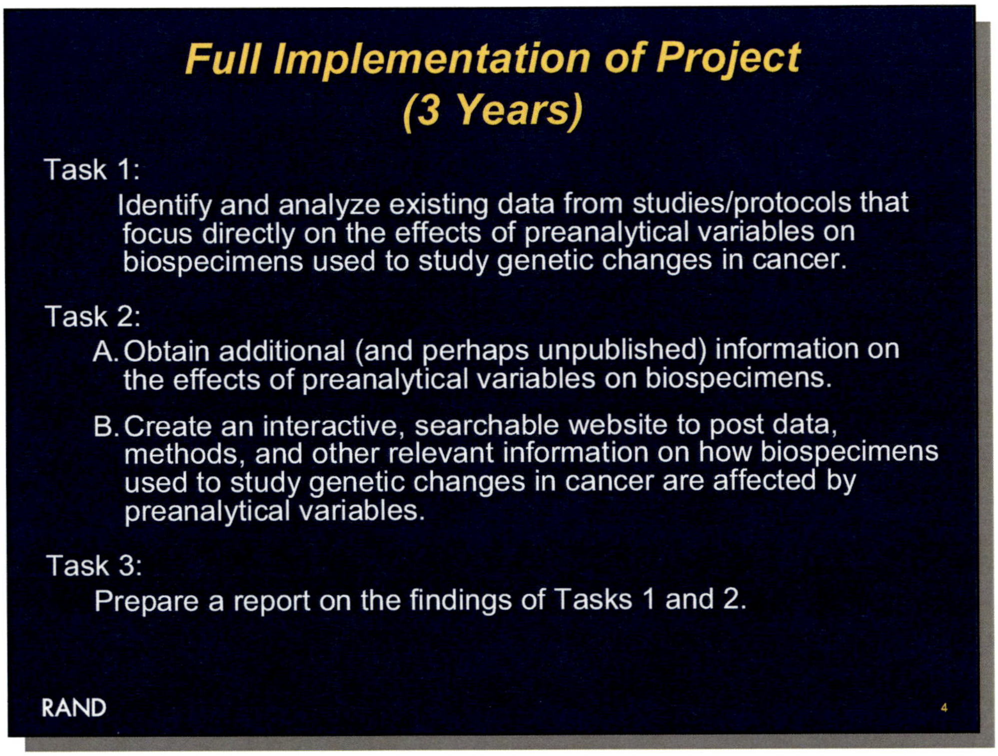

The full implementation of this project was envisioned as consisting of three tasks, which would be performed over a three-year period. The three tasks and associated subtasks are as follows:

TASK 1

Identify and analyze existing data from studies or protocols that focus directly on the effects of preanalytical variables on biospecimens used to study genetic and proteomic changes in cancer.

A. Conduct a comprehensive search of the scientific literature for studies done specifically to determine the effects of preanalytical variables on the quality of biospecimens used to study genetic and proteomic changes in cancer.

B. Review procedures for clinical laboratory testing relevant to research on genetic and proteomic changes in cancer (e.g., genetic testing, cytogenetics, molecular pathology) for data on the effects of preanalytical variables on the quality of biospecimens used to study genetic and proteomic changes in cancer.

TASK 2

A. Obtain additional (and perhaps unpublished) information on the effects of preanalytical variables on biospecimens.

- Conduct a comprehensive search of the scientific literature for studies that address preanalytical effects as part of the methodology section of the paper.

- Examine information about products used to collect, process, store, transport, and analyze biospecimens (e.g., DNA and RNA purification kits, DNA sequencers, real-time PCR machines) for information on the effects of preanalytical variables on biospecimens used to study genetic and proteomic changes in cancer.

- Request information from the scientific community about the effects of preanalytical variables on biospecimens used to study genetic and proteomic changes in cancer.

B. Create an interactive, searchable Web site to post data, methods, and other relevant information on how biospecimens used to study genetic and proteomic changes in cancer are affected by preanalytical variables.

TASK 3

Prepare a report on the findings of tasks 1 and 2.

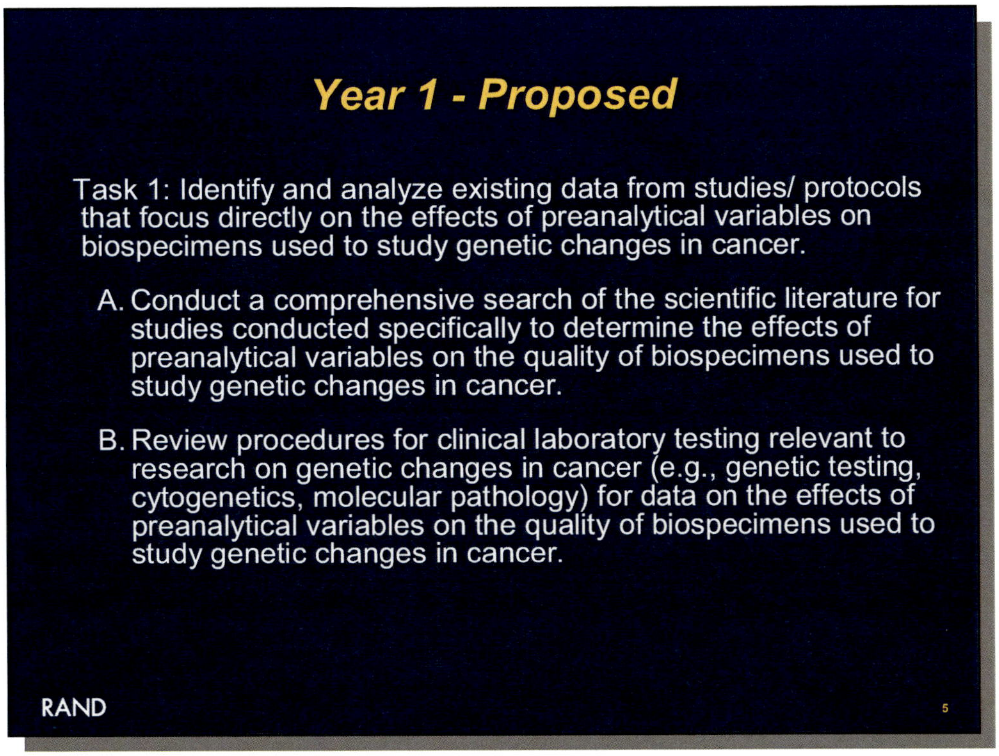

The project was broken down into three one-year intervals. The work proposed for year 1 of this project covered activities and requirements of task 1, with the possibility of subsequent tasks being added later as funding and priorities allow. Task 1 involves identifying and analyzing existing data from studies and protocols that focus directly on the effects of preanalytical variables on biospecimens used to study genetic and proteomic changes in cancer. Task 1 consists of two parts: (a) conducting a comprehensive search of the scientific literature for studies done specifically to determine the effects of preanalytical variables on the quality of biospecimens used to study genetic and proteomic changes in cancer and (b) reviewing procedures for clinical laboratory testing relevant to research on genetic and proteomic changes in cancer (e.g., genetic testing, cytogenetics, molecular pathology) to identify data on the effects of preanalytical variables on the quality of biospecimens used to study genetic and proteomic changes in cancer.

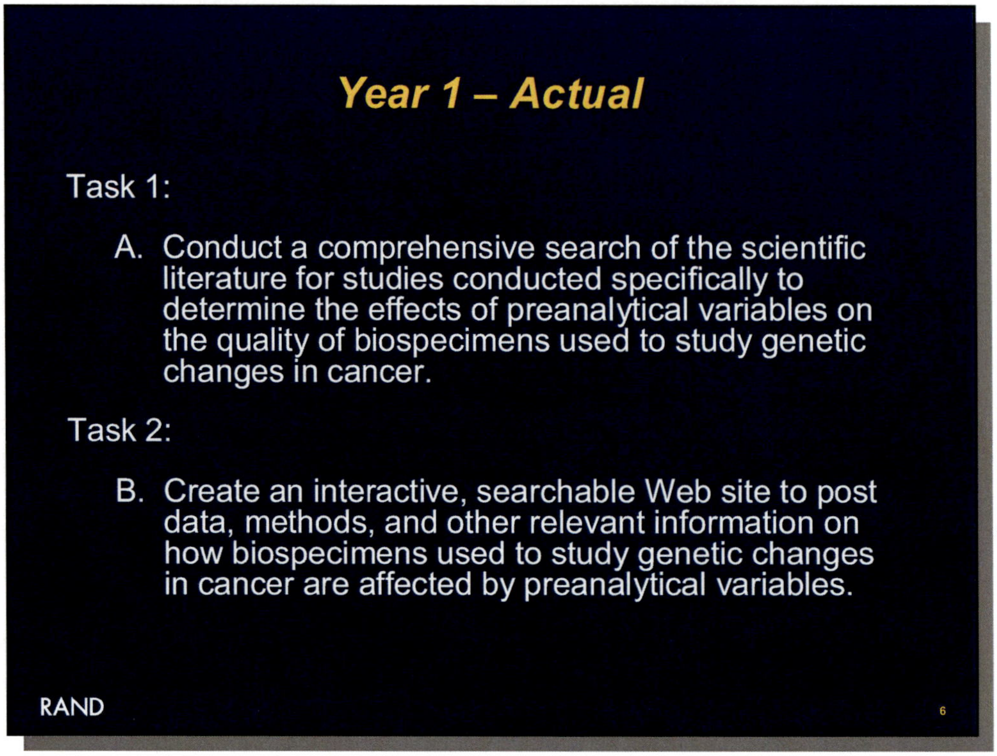

The work actually conducted during year 1 of the project, which is the focus of this documented briefing, was amended from what was originally proposed. OBBR and RAND realized that it would be advantageous to have the data collected during the review of the scientific literature available in a format that was easily accessible and searchable. Therefore, it was decided that it was more practical to begin the development of an interactive, searchable Web site during year 1 of the project instead of waiting until subsequent years. To accomplish this, task 2B was added to the work conducted during year 1:

> Task 2B: Create an interactive, searchable Web site to post data, methods, and other relevant information on how biospecimens used to study genetic and proteomic changes in cancer are affected by preanalytical variables.

The focus of task 2B was the development of an online data-collection Web site in collaboration with OBBR. The data-collection Web site was to be designed in such a way that, as data are entered, they directly populate an online, searchable database. The data-collection Web site and the eventual searchable database of the effects of preanalytical variables on the quality of biospecimens was to be built by OBBR with input from RAND and hosted on the OBBR external Web site.

Task 1 was amended so that the focus was solely on Task 1A, which entails conducting a comprehensive search of the scientific literature for studies done specifically to determine the effects of preanalytical variables on the quality of biospecimens used to study genetic and proteomic changes in cancer. Task 1B, which involves reviewing procedures for clinical laboratory testing relevant to research on genetic and proteomic changes in cancer for data on the effects of preanalytical variables, was postponed and not addressed during year 1.

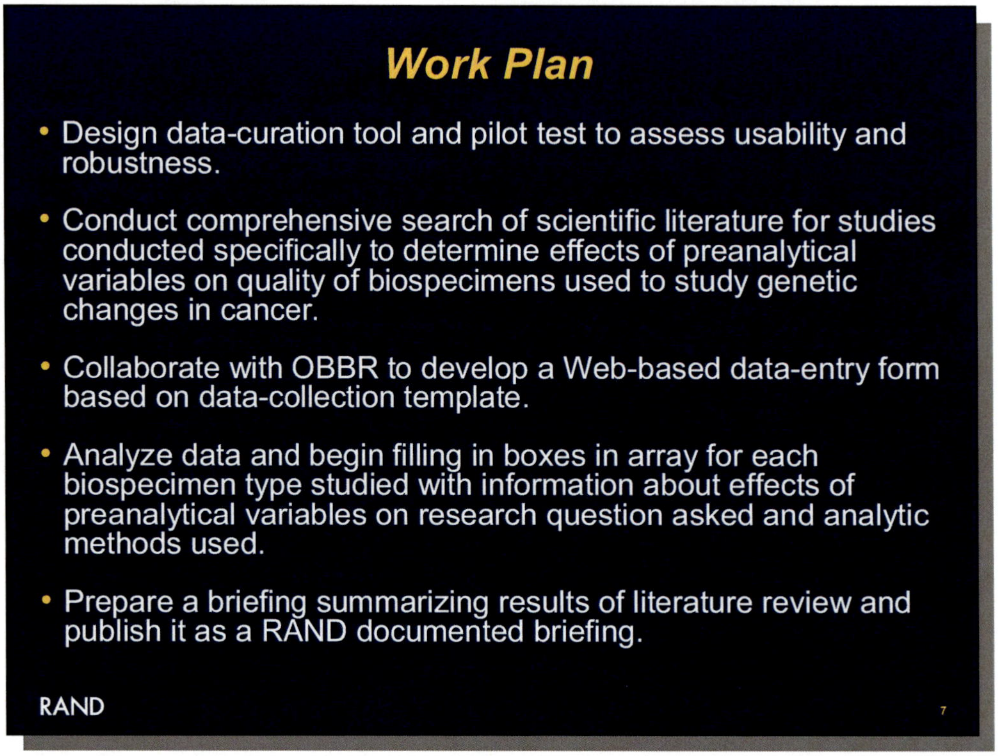

The work plan for the project included several steps. The first step was to design a data-curation tool and pilot test the tool to assess its usability and robustness. Once the data-curation tool was developed, a comprehensive search of the scientific literature would be performed to identify studies conducted specifically to determine the effects of preanalytical variables on the quality of biospecimens used to study genetic and proteomic changes in cancer. Information from papers selected through the literature search would be entered into the data-curation tool. A Web-based version of the data-curation tool would be developed in collaboration with OBBR. Data collected using the curation tool would be analyzed for each biospecimen type studied for information about the effects of preanalytical variable on the research question asked and the analytic methods used. Finally, a briefing summarizing the results of the literature review and the development of the data-curation tool would be presented to OBBR, and the briefing would be published as a RAND documented briefing.

The remainder of this documented briefing is organized as follows. Chapter Two describes the process of developing the data-curation tool, which serves as the basis of the Biospecimen Research Database. Chapter Three provides details on the review of the scientific literature to identify studies on the effects of preanalytical variables on biospecimens. Chapter Four presents the results of the study. The last chapter, Chapter Five, details some of the challenges encountered during the data analysis and presents next steps to expand the information in the Biospecimen Research Database.

CHAPTER TWO. DEVELOPING THE DATA-CURATION TOOL

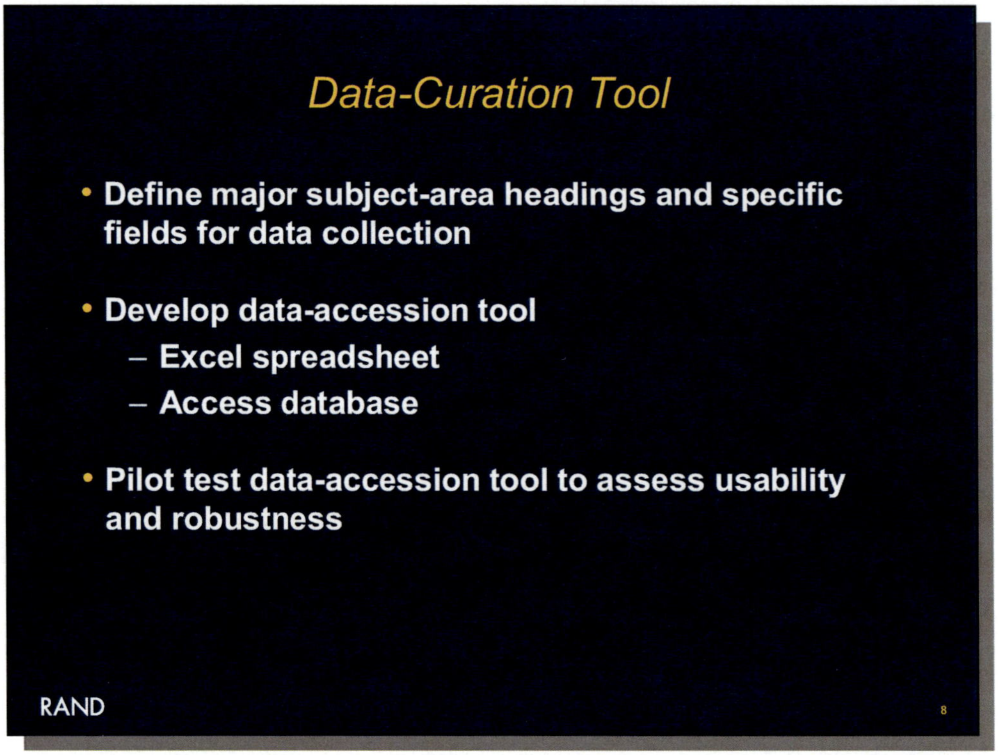

To make the findings of this project useful to the scientific community, it was necessary to develop a systematic way of capturing the wealth of data collected through the review of the scientific literature. A data-curation tool was developed to provide a standardized way of consistently recording data obtained through the literature review. Developing the data-curation tool involved several activities. First, the major subject-area headings and specific fields for data collection had to be defined. Next, a data-accession tool needed to be designed. A preliminary template was designed using a Microsoft Excel spreadsheet, which was pilot tested to determine whether the appropriate data-collection fields had been selected. A more user-friendly, interactive data-accession tool was then designed using a Microsoft Access database, which was also pilot tested to assess its usability and robustness. Each of these steps is described in more detail in the following slides.

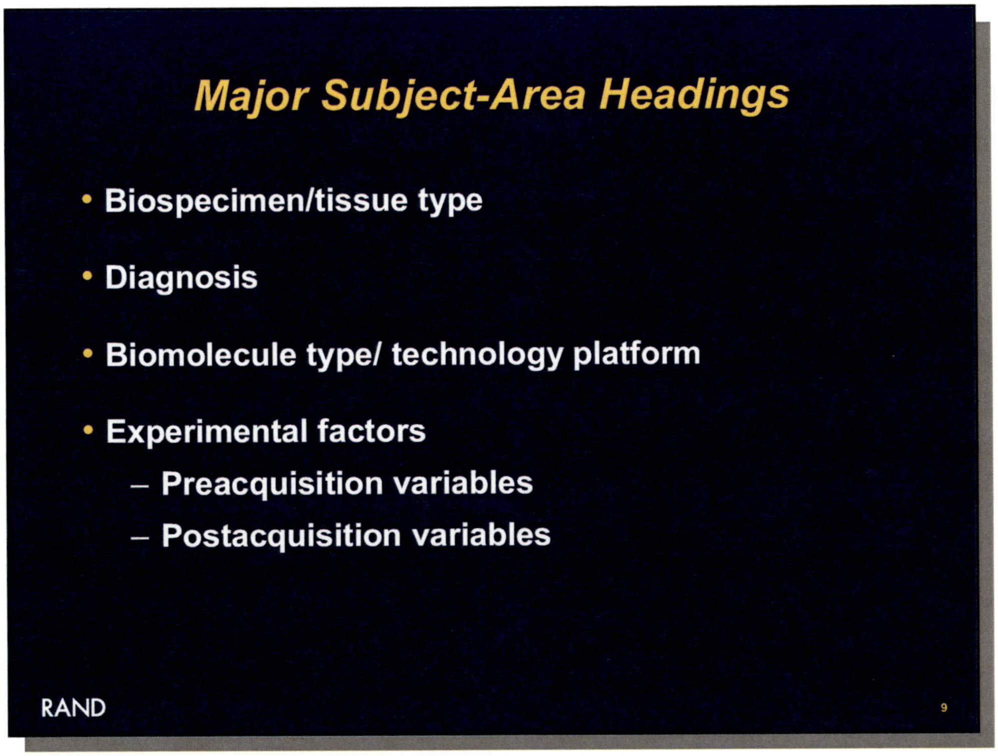

The first step in developing the data-curation tool was to determine the types of data that would be collected from the literature review. The types of data to be collected were grouped into major subject areas of interest. The major subject-area headings selected were as follows:

- biospecimen type: identifies the physical state of the biospecimen as *cell*, *tissue*, or *fluid*.
- tissue type: identifies the specific tissue from which the biospecimen was derived (e.g., brain, breast, lung, prostate)
- diagnosis: identifies the disease state of the tissue from which the biospecimen was derived; includes normal tissue, neoplastic tissue, and any of a number of other types of diseases and disorders, such as Alzheimer's disease, diabetes, hepatitis, multiple sclerosis, and rheumatoid arthritis
- biomolecule type: defines the biomolecule that will be studied as part of the research question (e.g., DNA, RNA, protein)
- technology platform: describes the method used to analyze the biomolecule of interest (e.g., PCR, cDNA microarrays, mass spectrometry)

- experimental factors (i.e., preanalytical variables): includes both preacquisition and postacquisition variables
- purpose of study: describes the focus and rationale for the study
- findings/conclusion of study: provides details about the results and conclusions of the study.

The next step was to identify specific fields for data collection within each major subject-area heading. Finally, relationships between the major subject areas were identified. It was decided that each biospecimen type was logically associated with certain tissue types. Once the biospecimen type was chosen, only the specific tissue types associated with that biospecimen type would be available for selection. It was also decided that the biomolecule type dictated which technology platform could be selected for its analysis. Therefore, biomolecule type and technology platform were combined into a single major subject-area heading.

The major subject-area headings and associated specific data-entry fields went through several revisions during the development of the Excel and Access data-curation tools. The major subject headings and associated specific data-entry fields were fine-tuned even more during the development of the Web-based, searchable database.[4] For example, the major subject-area heading originally titled "Tissue Type" is now called "Biospecimen Location" in the Web-based version of the database, and "Biomolecule" is now called "Analyte." In addition, new, specific data-entry fields have been added to the drop-down menus for "Technology Platform" and "Analyte." The Biospecimen Research Database was designed in such a way that it is relatively easy to make additional changes to the specific data-entry fields to accommodate the types of data found in the literature. The version used in the final Access data-curation tool is presented in the following slides.

---

[4] The Biospecimen Research Database is available to search online (OBBR, undated[d]).

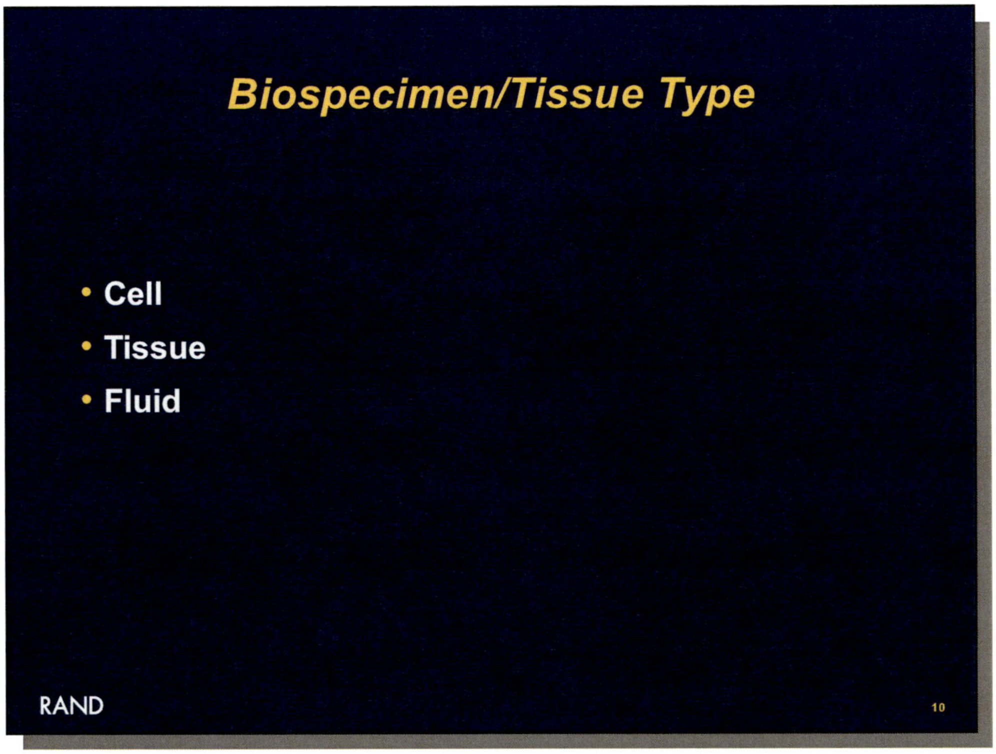

As mentioned earlier, biospecimen type and tissue type are closely related. The biospecimen type identifies the physical state of the biospecimen as *cell*, *tissue*, or *fluid*, while the tissue type identifies the specific tissue from which the biospecimen was derived (e.g., blood, brain, colon, lung, prostate). For example, if the biospecimen type is *fluid*, the tissue type would be limited to fluids within the body (e.g., amniotic fluid, blood, saliva, urine). Since each biospecimen type is logically associated with certain tissue types, the data-curation tool was designed in such a way that, once the biospecimen type was chosen, only the specific tissue types associated with that biospecimen type would be available for selection.

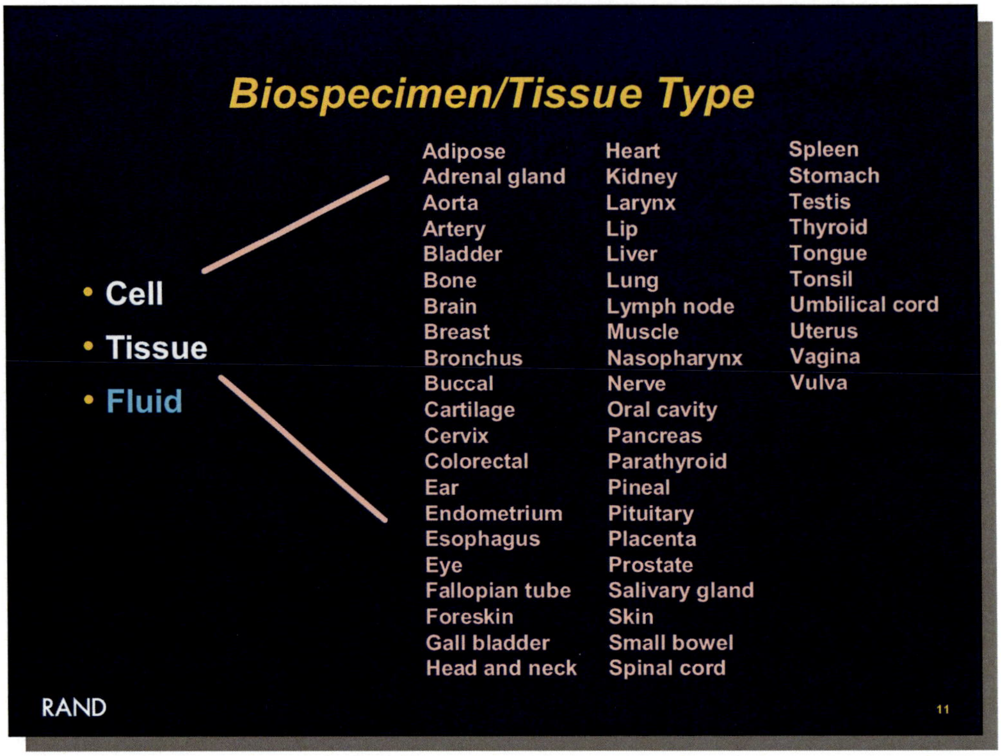

Cells and tissue can be derived from the same tissue types in the body. Therefore, the tissue types associated with the biospecimen types of *cell* and *tissue* are the same. In other words, whether *cell* or *tissue* is selected as the biospecimen type, the same list of tissue types will be available in the data-curation tool. For example, a sample from a breast biopsy would be a biospecimen type of *tissue*. However, if that breast biopsy was made into an immortalized cell line, the biospecimen type would be *cell*. Listed on this slide are many of the tissue types associated with the biospecimen types of *cell* and *tissue*, ranging from aorta, brain, and endometrium to prostate, skin, and uterus.

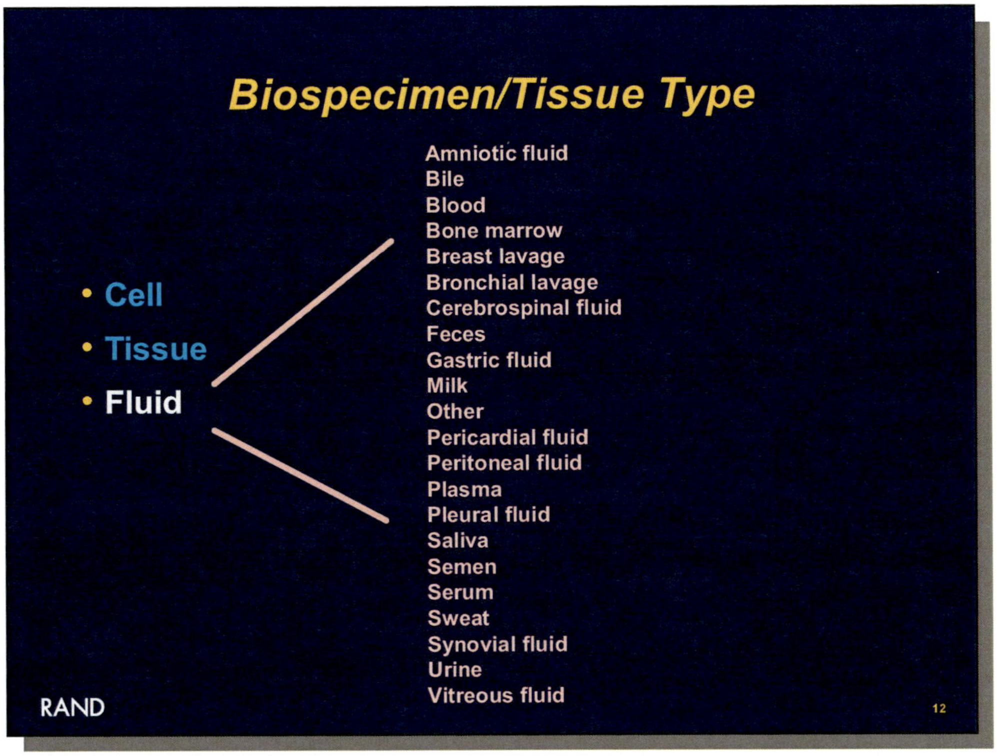

If the biospecimen type is *fluid*, the tissue type would be limited to fluids within the body (e.g., amniotic fluid, blood, saliva, urine). This slide shows the many tissue types associated with the biospecimen type of *fluid*, including amniotic fluid, blood, bone marrow, cerebrospinal fluid, plasma, saliva, and urine. There is also the choice of "Other," which can be selected for other types of fluids that are not found on the list.

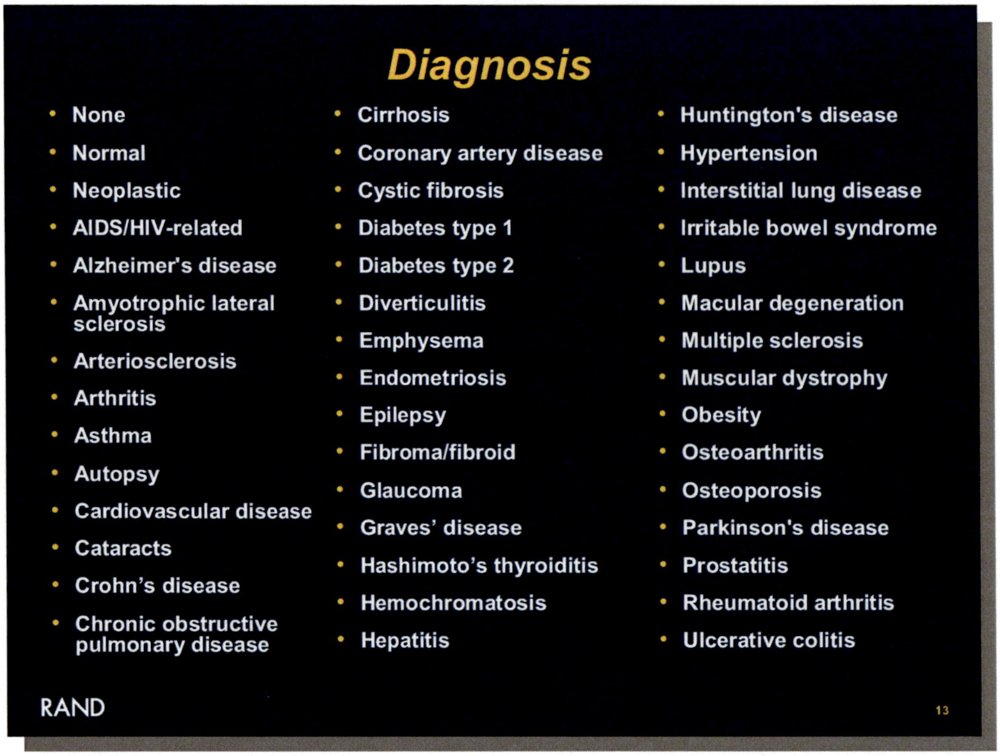

The diagnosis major subject area identifies the disease state of the tissue from which the biospecimen was derived. If the biospecimen comes from a tissue that is not diseased, then "Normal" would be selected for the diagnosis. Studies sometimes indicate only that the biospecimens were obtained during an autopsy, without any information on the cause of death or the disease state of the tissue. For these studies, "Autopsy" would be selected for the diagnosis. Sometimes, studies do not indicate the disease state of the tissue. For these studies, "None" would be selected for the diagnosis.

The diagnosis of *neoplastic* includes biospecimens from all types of cancer, as well as benign tumors and tissue just adjacent to the neoplasm. Because neoplastic biospecimens can represent very different diseases, the diagnosis of *neoplastic* was divided up into subcategories, which are described in more detail in the next slide.

Several other types of diseases and disorders can also be selected, such as Alzheimer's disease, diabetes, hepatitis, multiple sclerosis, and rheumatoid arthritis. However, since the focus of this project was on the effects of preanalytical variables on biospecimens used for cancer research, none of the studies analyzed utilized biospecimens with these other diagnoses.

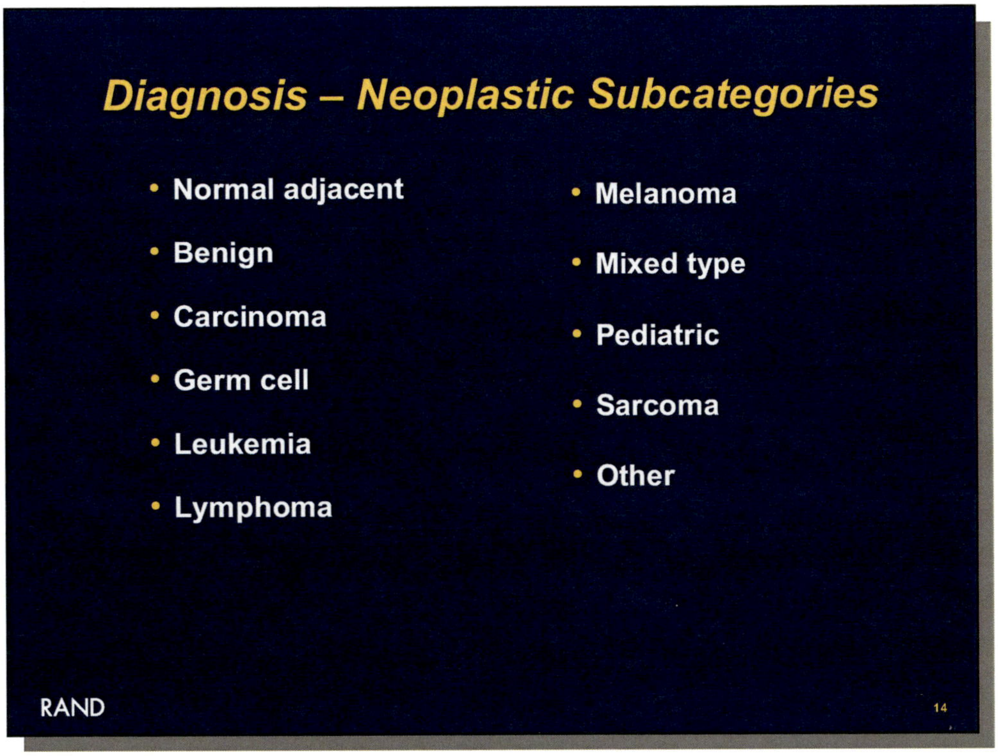

Neoplastic biospecimens can come from patients with very different kinds of diseases, including more than 100 types of cancer (e.g., breast cancer, prostate cancer, chronic lymphocytic leukemia, melanoma), as well as benign tumors (e.g., moles, uterine fibroids, lipomas, pituitary adenomas). To allow for a more accurate characterization of the specific diagnosis for neoplastic biospecimens, the diagnosis of *neoplastic* was divided up into several subcategories.

Instead of listing every type of cancer in an exhaustive list, cancer types were grouped into broader categories, including carcinoma, germ cell, leukemia, lymphoma, melanoma, mixed type, pediatric, and sarcoma. The choice of "Other" was also included for other types of neoplastic tissues that are not found on the list. Because benign tumors are not cancerous, the subcategory "Benign" was also included. Tissue just adjacent to the neoplasm (i.e., normal adjacent tissue) is not typically considered to be neoplastic, but it is not considered to be normal either. Therefore, "Normal Adjacent" was included as a selection in the neoplastic subcategories.

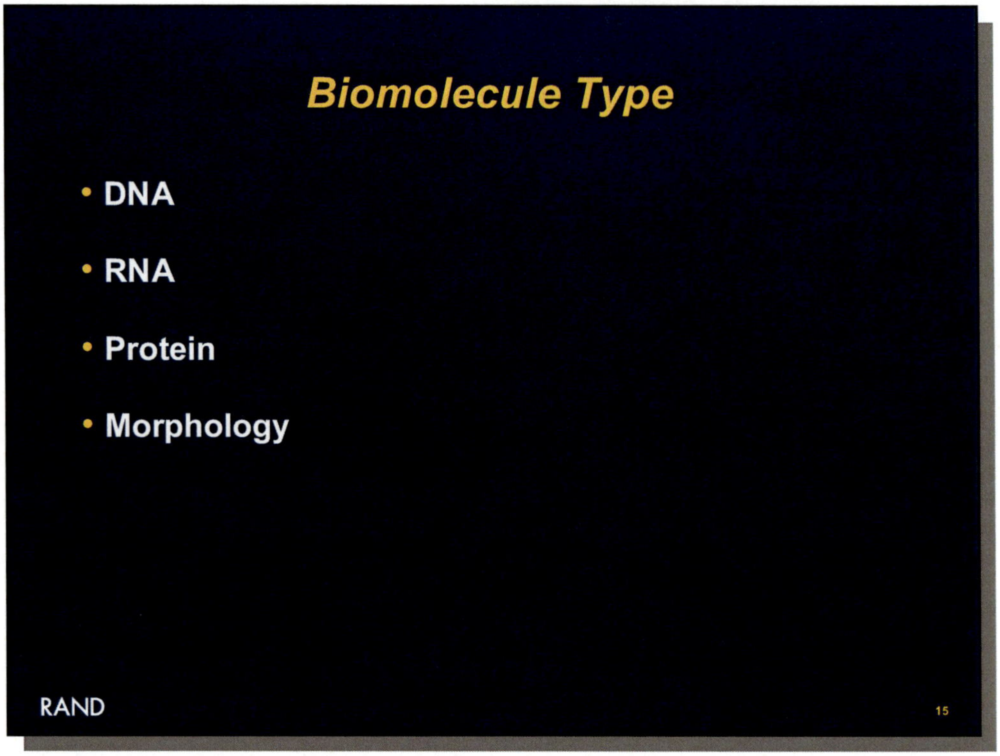

The biomolecule type defines the biomolecule that will be studied as part of the research question. The three main biomolecules of interest for studying the genetic and proteomic changes in cancer are DNA, RNA, and protein. These are also the biomolecules within the cell that are most commonly altered by exposure to preanalytical variables. The biomolecule type also dictates which technology platform will be selected for its analysis. Therefore, biomolecule type and technology platform were combined into a single major subject-area heading.

Although *morphology* is not a biomolecule type, for the purposes of developing the data-curation tool, it was grouped together with DNA, RNA, and protein under the major subject-area heading of "Biomolecule Type."[5] The rational for this grouping and the technology platforms associated with each biomolecule type are described in the following slides.

---

[5] *Morphology* is the study of the size, shape, and structure of a particular organism, organ, tissue, or cell. For the purposes of this documented briefing, the term *morphology* refers to the examination of the detailed structure of cells and tissues (sometimes called cellular morphology). Techniques used to study the morphology of cells and tissues include histology, immunohistochemistry, in situ hybridization, electron microscopy, and light, fluorescent, and confocal microscopy.

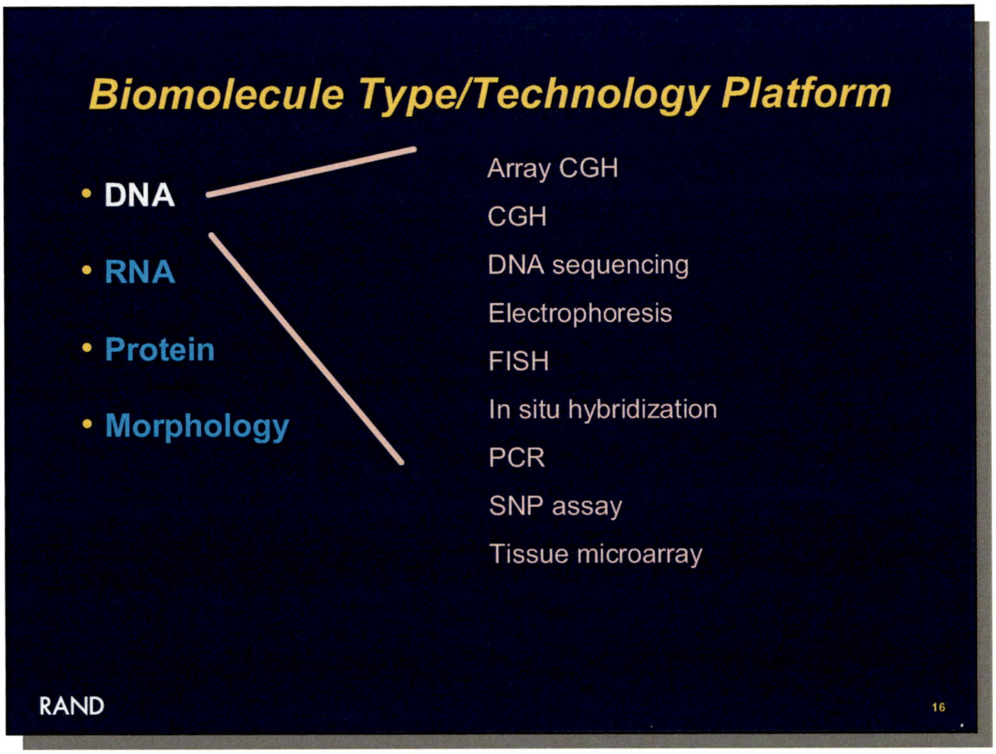

The technology platform describes the method used to analyze the biomolecule of interest. Each biomolecule type can be analyzed using a set of assays specific to that biomolecule type. The final data-curation tool was designed so that the biomolecule type and the specific technology platforms associated with that biomolecule type were linked.

DNA can be analyzed using several different technology platforms. The most commonly used techniques to analyze DNA include comparative genomic hybridization (CGH), sequencing, electrophoresis, fluorescent in situ hybridization (FISH), PCR, single nucleotide polymorphism (SNP) assay, and tissue microarrays.

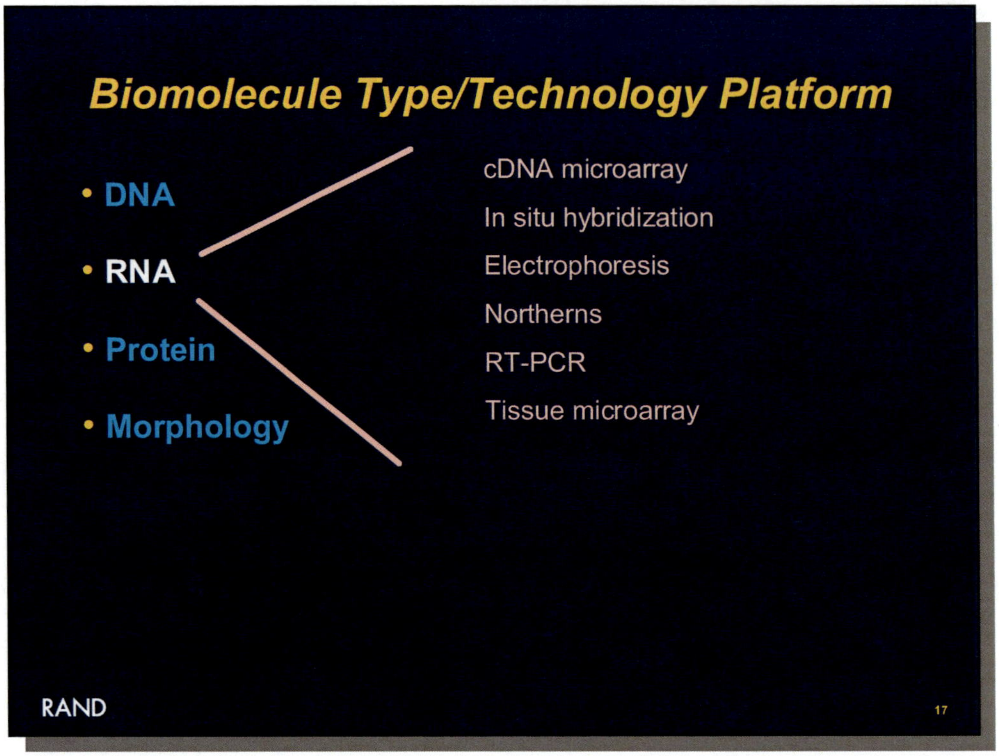

RNA can be analyzed using several different technology platforms. The most commonly used techniques to analyze RNA include cDNA microarrays, in situ hybridization, electrophoresis, Northern blots, reverse transcription PCR (RT-PCR), real-time PCR, and tissue microarrays.

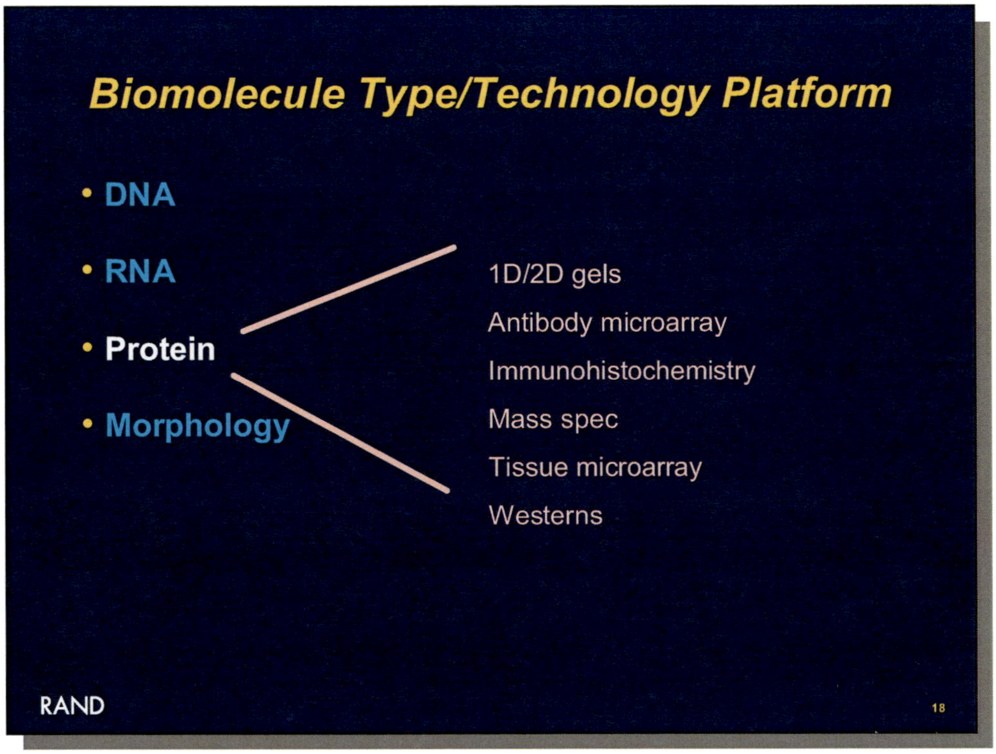

Protein can be analyzed using several different technology platforms. The most commonly used techniques to analyze protein are one- and two-dimensional (1D and 2D, respectively) gel electrophoresis, antibody and tissue microarrays, immunohistochemistry, mass spectrometry, and Western blots.

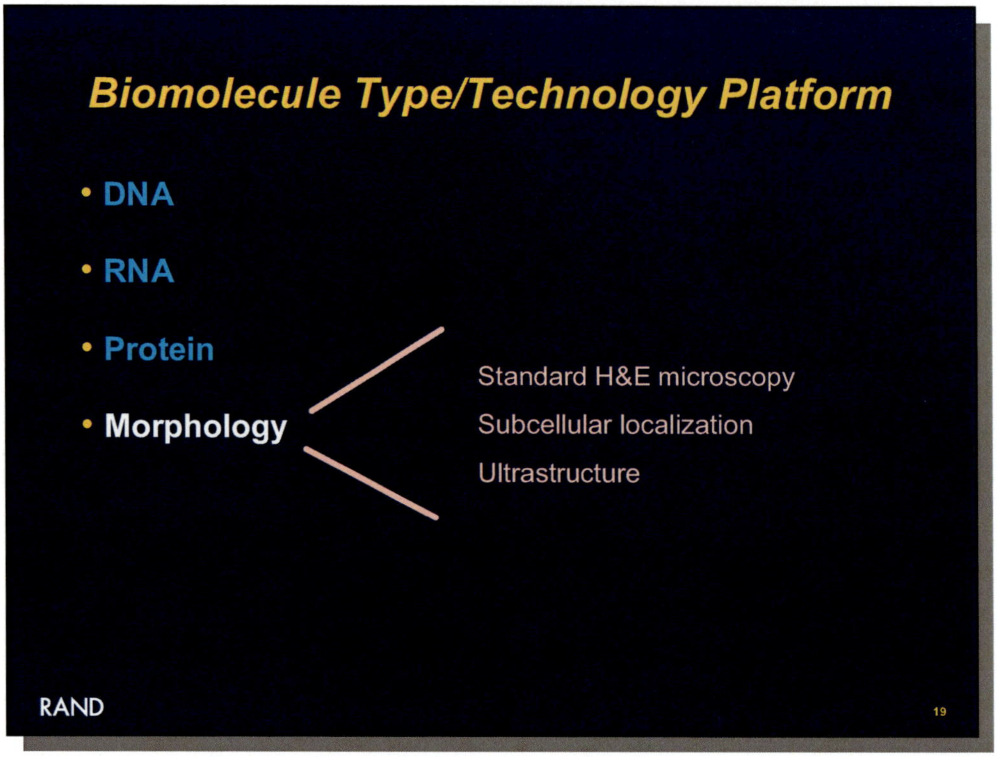

Morphology was grouped together with DNA, RNA, and protein under the major subject-area heading of "Biomolecule Type." The rationale behind this categorization is based on a few factors. First, analysis of DNA, RNA, or protein provides information at the molecular level about the impact of a disease or the effects of preanalytical variables on a biospecimen, while morphological analysis provides a broad indication of changes that may have occurred. For example, a biospecimen may show morphological changes consistent with necrosis, which may be due to an advanced stage of cancer or to the fact that the biospecimen was fixed in such a way that the overall structural integrity of the biospecimen was compromised. In addition, when a biospecimen is processed to isolate the biomolecule of interest, it is important to preserve both the integrity of the specimen for pathologic diagnosis and the biomolecule for molecular diagnosis. Therefore, many of preanalytical variables may have an effect on both morphology and the biomolecule being studied. A few specific technology platforms associated with *morphology* include standard hematoxylin and eosin (H&E) morphology, subcellular localization, and ultrastructure.

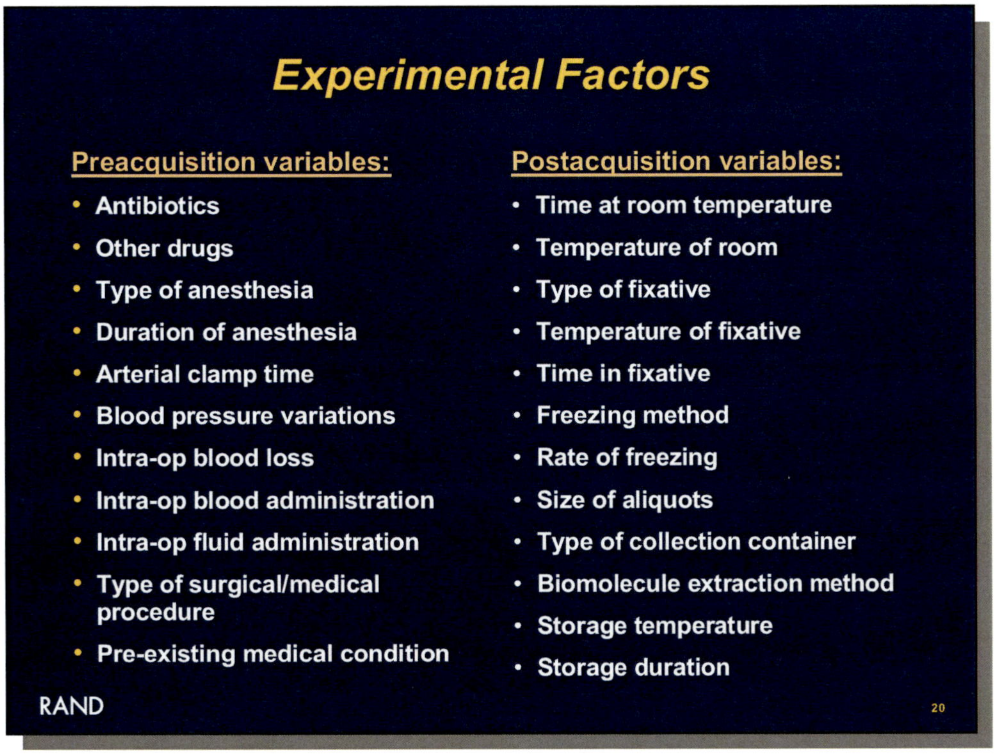

Preanalytical variables, captured under the major subject-area heading of "Experimental Factors," can be divided up into preacquisition and postacquisition variables. Preacquisition variables are conditions that occur any time before the actual biospecimen collection. Examples of preacquisition variables include physiological responses to antibiotics or other medications, the type and duration of anesthesia given during surgery, blood pressure variations during surgery, intraoperative blood or fluid administration, and the type of surgical or medical procedure performed. Postacquisition variables are conditions that occur from the time the biospecimen is collected up until the time it is used by the researcher for experimental purposes. Examples of postacquisition variables include the time a biospecimen sits at room temperature once it is removed, the type of fixative that is used, the method and rate of freezing, the size of the aliquots, the storage temperature and duration, and the method used to extract the biomolecule of interest.

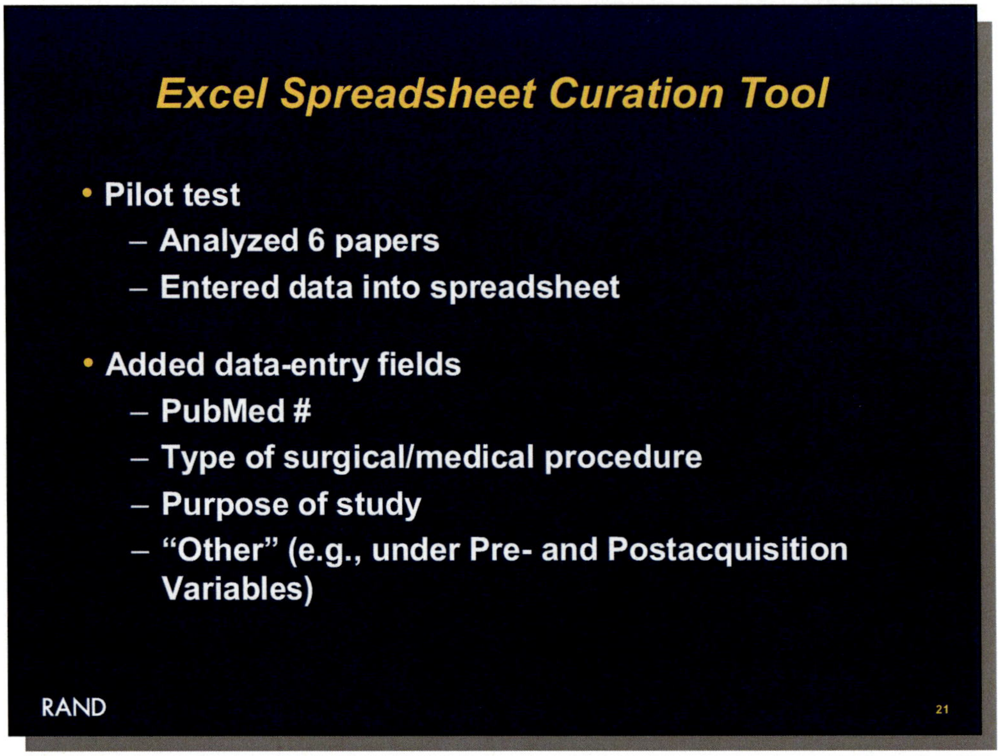

The data-collection template was developed to facilitate collection and analysis of information found during the review of the scientific literature. A preliminary template was designed using an Excel spreadsheet. The Excel data-collection template contained the major subject-area headings similar to the ones described earlier, but the data-entry fields and associations between major subject areas had not yet been finalized.

The Excel data-collection template was tested and refined by conducting a pilot test. The pilot test consisted of reviewing six peer-reviewed journal articles and using the template as a way to collect and organize the data. All six papers were reviewed by three people, and the results of the reviews were compared for consistency. Pilot testing the data-collection template in this way allowed a test of the usability and robustness of the template. It also allowed the template to be refined by the addition and deletion of data-entry fields based on the type and importance of information found in the papers.

Based on this pilot test, a few other fields were added to the template. The PubMed number was added as part of the paper identification information and to aid in retrieval of references by those using the database. The type of surgical or medical procedure was added as a postacquisition variable. A field to enter the purpose of the study was added so that visitors to the database could easily determine which studies were of interest. The choice of "Other" was also included for both preacquisition and postacquisition variables for other types of variables that are not found on the lists.

Details about the design and content of the Excel data-collection template are presented in the next two slides.

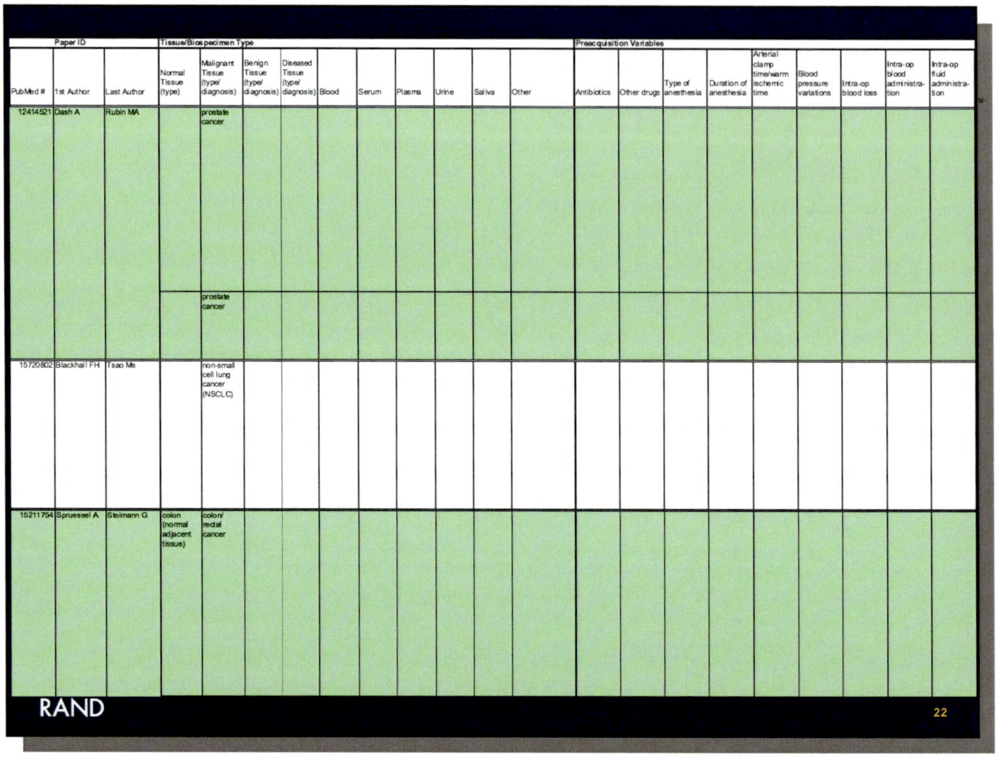

Paper ID			Tissue/Biospecimen Type									
PubMed #	1st Author	Last Author	Normal Tissue (type)	Malignant Tissue (type/ diagnosis)	Benign Tissue (type/ diagnosis)	Diseased Tissue (type/ diagnosis)	Blood	Serum	Plasma	Urine	Saliva	Other
12414521	Dash A	Rubin MA		prostate cancer								
				prostate cancer								
15720802	Blackhall FH	Tsao Ms		non-small cell lung cancer (NSCLC)								
15211754	Spruessel A	Steimann G	colon (normal adjacent tissue)	colon/ rectal cancer								

Paper ID	Preacquisition Variables								
PubMed #	Antibiotics	Other drugs	Type of anesthesia	Duration of anesthesia	Arterial clamp time/warm ischemic time	Blood pressure variations	Intra-op blood loss	Intra-op blood administra-tion	Intra-op fluid administra-tion
12414521									
15720802									
15211754									

The Excel data-collection template shown here contains data from the pilot test. The major subject-area headings and specific data-entry fields are arrayed across the top of the spreadsheet. The template is so large that only some of the data-entry columns are shown on this slide and the next slide. The far left of the slide shows that each paper reviewed was identified by its PubMed number and first and last author. Next, the tissue or biospecimen type and preacquisition variables were entered.

Because the Excel template was used early on in the development of the data-curation tool, the major subject-area headings and specific data-entry fields differ a bit from the final ones presented here. The major subject-area headings and data-entry fields in the Excel data-collection template were

- Tissue/Biospecimen Type
    - Normal Tissue (type)
    - Malignant Tissue (type/diagnosis)
    - Benign Tissue (type/diagnosis)
    - Diseased Tissue (type/diagnosis)
    - Blood
    - Serum
    - Plasma
    - Urine

- Saliva
- Other

- Preacquisition Variables
  - Antibiotics
  - Other drugs
  - Type of anesthesia
  - Duration of anesthesia
  - Arterial clamp time/warm ischemic time
  - Blood pressure variations
  - Intra-op blood loss
  - Intra-op blood administration
  - Intra-op fluid administration
  - Type of surgical/medical procedure
  - Pre-existing medical conditions
  - Patient gender
  - Other
- Postacquisition Variables
  - Time at room temperature/pre-fixation time
  - Temperature of room
  - Type of fixative
  - Temperature of fixative
  - Time in fixative
  - Freezing method
  - Rate of freezing
  - Size of specimen aliquots
  - Type of collection container
  - Biomolecule extraction method
  - Storage temperature
  - Storage duration
  - Storage in vacuum
  - Other
- Morphological Analysis
  - Standard H&E microscopy
  - Immunohistochemistry
  - Ultrastructure
  - Subcellular localization
  - FISH
  - Tissue Microarrays
  - In situ hybridization
  - Other
- Biomolecule Type
  - DNA

- RNA
    - Protein
    - Other
- Technology Platform
    - PCR
    - DNA Sequencing
    - SNP assay
    - Comparative Genomic Hybridization (CGH)
    - RT-PCR
    - Northern blots
    - cDNA Microarrays
    - Mass Spectroscopy
    - Western blots
    - 1D/2D protein gels
    - Other
- Purpose of Study
- Findings/Conclusions of Study

There are some differences in the major subject-area headings and specific data-entry fields between the Excel data-entry template and the final Access database curation tool worth noting. The first is the way in which the specific data-entry fields under the heading Tissue/Biospecimen Type are set up in the Excel template. Instead of having all of the possible tissue types listed, Tissue/Biospecimen is broken down into Normal Tissue, Malignant Tissue, Benign Tissue, and Diseased Tissue, and the curator is asked to enter the type of tissue and the diagnosis (i.e., where "(type/diagnosis)" is indicated next to each of these headings) into the appropriate cell in the Excel spreadsheet. For example, for the first study by Dash et al. (2002), the Tissue/Biospecimen Type was "Malignant Tissue" and the "type/diagnosis" was "prostate cancer." "Blood," "Serum," "Plasma," "Urine," "Saliva," and "Other" are also listed. Also, the breakdown by cell, tissue, and fluid, as explained earlier, was not present. The other difference between the Excel data-entry template and the final Access database curation tool is that "Morphological Analysis" is its own major subject-area heading in the Excel template instead of being grouped with Biomolecule Type like it is in the final Access database curation tool.

While conducting the pilot test, it became evident that individual papers could contain information about multiple studies, each with its own purpose and findings. For example, a paper looking at the effects of different fixation methods may contain three studies that address different aspects of the main question, such as (1) a study looking at the effects of fixation on the quality of DNA using PCR, (2) a study looking at the effects of fixation on the expression of certain genes using cDNA microarrays, and (3) a study looking at the effects of fixation on morphology of the biospecimen using standard H&E microscopy. Therefore, it was decided that data would be entered at the level of each individual study instead at the level of the entire paper. Shown on this slide are data entered from three papers representing four studies—the first paper, by Dash et al. (2002) (highlighted in green at the top of the slide), contains two studies, and the second paper, by Blackhall et al. (2004) (in white), contains only one study. The last paper, by Spruessel et al. (2004) (highlighted in green at the bottom of the slide), actually has two studies, but only one is shown on the slide.

Technology Platform											Purpose of Study	Findings/Conclusions of Study	Reference	
PCR	DNA Sequenc-ing	SNP assay	Comparative Genomic Hybridization (CGH)	RT-PCR	Northerns	cDNA Micro-arrays	Mass Spec	Westerns	1D/2D protein gels	Other			Pub Med Link	Publication Year
						Research Genetics human cDNA clone set, 4400 ESTs					To study the increase in gene expression and identify individual genes that may be artifacts of processing of prostate tissue obtained from radical prostactectomy specimens removed as treatment for localized prostate cancer.	Identified 61 statistically significant genes that were overexpressed after 1 hr at room temperature – 41 of which were named genes. Several of these genes are known to be early response gene, genes implicated in hypoxia, or transcription factors, including jun B proto-oncogene (JUNB), jun D proto-oncogene (JUND), and activating transcription factor 3 (ATF3). In contrast, expression of several genes implicated in prostate cancer development, e.g., hepsin, AMACR, fatty acid synthase, PTEN, and PIM-1, remained relatively constant. Early growth response 1 (EGR1), which has previously been shown to function as a master switch to activate several cellular responses to ischemic stress and has been shown to have increased expression has been previously associated with prostate cancer, had increased expression with increased incubation time at room temperature before processing. Therefore, processing time (i.e., time at room temperature before processing) may introduce artifacts into the gene expression profile for prostate tissue specimens.	http://www.ncbi.nlm.nih.gov/entrez/query.fcgi?db=pubmed&cmd=Retrieve&dopt=Abstract&list_uids=12414521&query_hl=14&itool=pubmed_docsum	2002
								EGR1			To confirm the increase in early growth response 1 (EGR1) protein expression that may be an artifact of processing of prostate tissue obtained from radical prostactectomy specimens removed as treatment for localized prostate cancer.	EGR1 protein expression increased with time that specimens sat at room temperature before being processed. Therefore, increased protein expression of EGR1 in prostate tissue specimens may be an artifact of processing time.		
				JNK3, JUN-B, AP-1, CAIX, PRSS25, HHR6B		University Health Network Microarray Centre (Canada) 1.7K clone set					To examine the effect of time on gene expression in tumor samples maintained at room temperature for different time periods following surgical resection of non small cell lung cancer before snap-freezing in liquid nitrogen.	When different samples of a tumor were snap-frozen at increasing time intervals following surgical resection, the quality of RNA did not deteriorate, and there was not a global decline in mean gene expression nor a clear pattern of change in relative gene expression with time. Expression of two genes was shown to have a linear relationship with time. In addition, significant heterogeneity existed in the expression levels of stress and hypoxia-activated genes in samples obtained from different areas of the same tumor specimen snap-frozen 30 minutes after resection. Variation due to heterogeneity within each tumor (i.e., between samples taken from multiple sites within a tumor) was significantly greater than variation due to time between resection and freezing. Samples snap-frozen within 30 to 60 minutes of surgical resection were acceptable for gene expression studies;	http://www.ncbi.nlm.nih.gov/entrez/query.fcgi?db=pubmed&cmd=Retrieve&dopt=Abstract&list_uids=15720802&query_hl=19&itool=pubmed_docsum	2004
				hypoxia-inducible factor 1(~ (HIF-1( ), c-fos, heme oxygenase 1 (HO-1), CK20, CEA		Affymetrix GeneChip HG-U133A					To determine the impact of ischemia on gene expression profiles of healthy and malignant colon tissue and, thus, on screening studies for identification of molecular targets and diagnostic molecular patterns.	No differences of RNA quality were observed over a period of 30 minutes. Changes in gene expression profiles were already observed 5-8 minutes after colon resection. 15 minutes after surgery, 10-15% of all genes differed significantly (>2-fold) from the baseline values, and by 30 minutes after surgery, 20% of all detectable genes differed. Significant changes of expression were found in known hypoxia-realted molecules (HIF-1(-and c-fos), as well as cytoskeletal genes (e.g., CK20) and tumor-associated antigens (e.g., CEA). Changes of expression were also found in molecules ina wide variety of functional groups, such as oncogenes, transduction, nuclear genes, kinases, chaperones, and cell growth. Therefore, preanalytical factors, such as tissue ischemia time, dramatically affect gene expression.	http://www.ncbi.nlm.nih.gov/entrez/query.fcgi?db=pubmed&cmd=Retrieve&dopt=Abstract&list_uids=15211754&query_hl=11&itool=pubmed_docsum	2004

Shown on this slide is another portion of the Excel template for the same three papers shown earlier. This portion of the Excel template is where the curator records information about the technology platform, the purpose of the study, and the findings or conclusion of the study. In addition, the full citation is recorded for each paper, including the publication year, authors, title, journal name, issue, and page numbers (not shown). A link to the PubMed abstract is also recorded, when available.

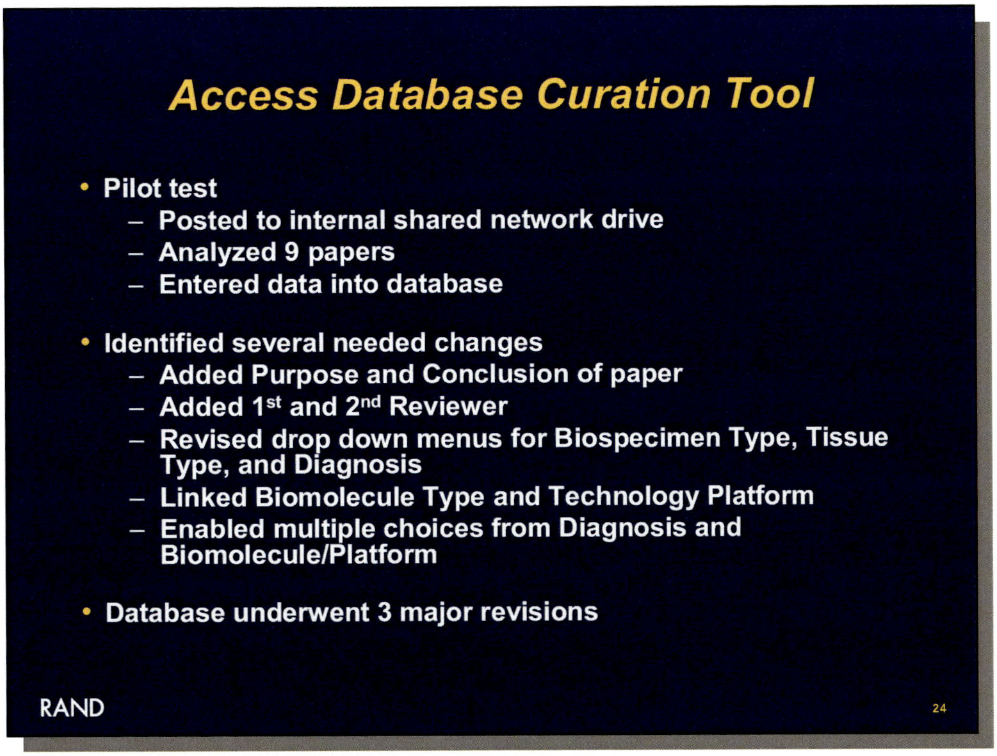

The Access database curation tool was developed in collaboration with OBBR. The fields defined in the Excel data-collection template formed the basis of the Access database curation tool. Data-entry forms with drop-down menus and free-text boxes were developed to improve the ease of data entry. Two different forms were developed: one to capture general information about the paper (i.e., "Papers") and one to capture specific data about the studies within the paper (i.e., "Studies").

The Access database curation tool was posted to an internal, shared network drive at RAND so that multiple curators could interact with it easily through the network. There was a master curator who had full access to the Access database curation tool to make changes in the forms and tables, and reviewers could enter data into the forms but could not make changes to the forms or tables. The database was password protected to establish these different levels of access. Data were entered and forms and reports were viewed, created, updated, or edited directly on the shared network drive according to the established levels of access.

The Access database curation tool was pilot tested. The pilot test consisted of entering data from the six papers analyzed during the pilot test of the Excel template plus three additional papers into the Access database. The pilot test of the Access database curation tool provided a direct comparison to the Excel template, confirmed its usability and robustness, and provided indications of where revisions of data-entry fields were necessary.

The database underwent three major revisions, with several changes made to the curation tool. Additional fields were added to the Papers form to record the overall purpose and conclusion of the paper. New fields were also added to the Papers form to track the reviewers of the papers. Each paper was reviewed by a primary reviewer and then checked for accuracy and completeness by a secondary reviewer.

On the Studies form, the drop-down menus for "Biospecimen Type" and "Tissue Type" were revised. Originally, these menus closely followed the major subject-area headings and specific data-entry fields used in the Excel template. Based on the pilot testing, the choices under "Biospecimen Type" were changed to *cell*, *tissue*, or *fluid*, and "Biospecimen Type" was linked to "Tissue Type" so that, once the biospecimen type was chosen, only the specific tissue types associated with that biospecimen type would be available for selection.

A new field called "Preservation" was also added to the Studies form. This field is used to record the method used to preserve the biospecimen, including fixatives (e.g., ethanol, formalin, optimum cutting temperature [OCT], embedding compound, RNAlater®), and other methods of preservation, such as flash freezing.

The drop-down menu for "Diagnosis" was also revised. All of the specific types of cancer (e.g., Hodgkin lymphoma, Kaposi sarcoma) were removed from the "Diagnosis" drop-down menu and replaced with the general term "Neoplastic." Then a "Diagnosis" subcategory, which grouped cancer types into broader categories, was added and linked to the diagnosis of "Neoplastic" to allow for a more accurate characterization of the diagnosis for neoplastic biospecimens. In addition, the ability to list several diagnoses was added so that studies conducted with of multiple types of biospecimens could be captured on the same form. For example, if a study was conducted using biospecimens from both colon cancer and normal adjacent tissue, both of those diagnoses could be entered on the same form.

Based on the pilot testing, "Biomolecule Type" and "Technology Platform" were combined into a single major subject-area heading on the Studies form. Instead of first choosing the biomolecule of interest (e.g., DNA, RNA, protein) from one drop-down menu and then choosing the corresponding technology platform from another drop-down menu, the choices in the drop-down menu were combined so that the biomolecule and technology platform appear together—e.g., "RNA/cDNA Microarray" instead of first choosing "RNA" from one menu and then choosing "cDNA Microarray" from the next menu (see the following slides for more details).

The Access database curation tool formed the basis for the development of an online data-collection Web site. The online data-collection Web site, which is still under development, was designed in such a way that, as data are entered, they directly populate an online, searchable database. The data-collection Web site and the searchable database of the effects of preanalytical variables on the quality of biospecimens is being built by OBBR with input from RAND and hosted on the OBBR external Web site. A prototype version is available online as a Web-based, searchable database that provides information about the effects of preanalytical variables on biospecimens.[6]

---

[6] The Biospecimen Research Database is available to search online (OBBR, undated [d]).

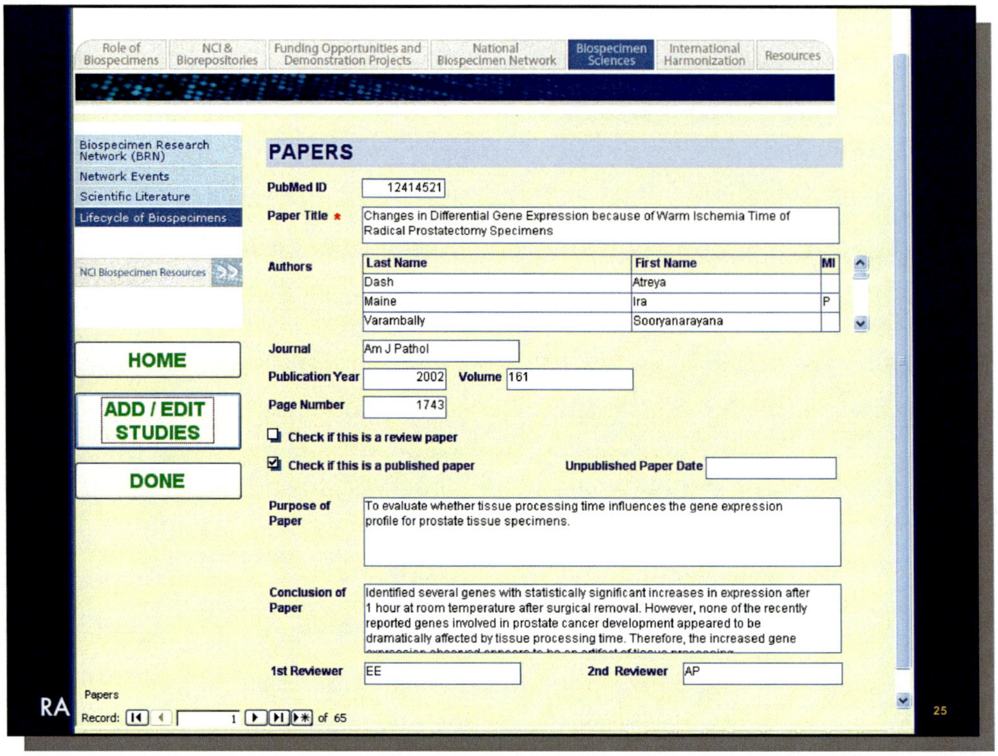

The Papers form provides data-entry fields to record general information about the paper, including the PubMed identification number, the title of the paper, authors' names, the journal name, volume, page number, and publication year. There is also a place to indicate whether the paper is a review article, a published paper, or an unpublished paper. The unpublished-paper field was included in anticipation of collecting data from unpublished research. There are free-text boxes to record the purpose and conclusion of the paper. Finally, there are boxes to record the initials of the first and second reviewers of the paper.

Clicking on the "Add/Edit Studies" button on the left side of the form takes the user to the Studies form, shown on the next two slides.

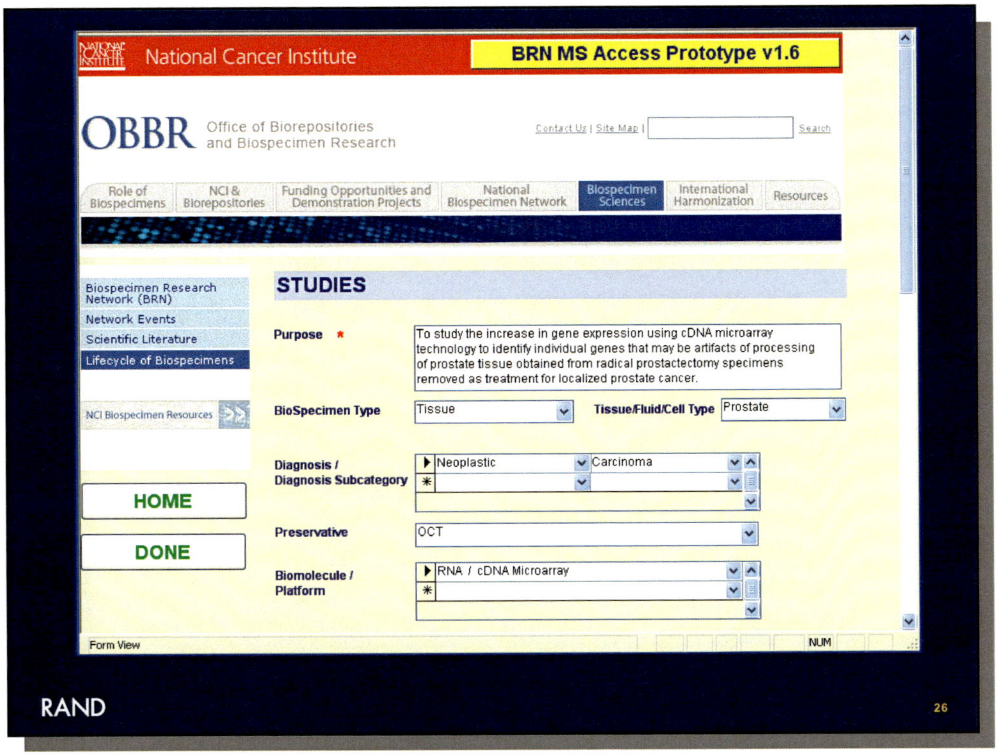

The Studies form provides data-entry fields to record specific data from the individual studies within a paper. The top half of the Studies form contains free-text boxes to record the purpose of the study and drop-down menus to record the biospecimen type, tissue, fluid or cell type, diagnosis, preservative, biomolecule, and technology platform. In the new "Biomolecule/Platform" drop-down menu, the choices from the old menus were combined so that the biomolecule and technology platform appear together:

- DNA/Array CGH
- DNA/CGH
- DNA/DNA Sequencing
- DNA/Electrophoresis
- DNA/FISH
- DNA/In situ hybridization
- DNA/PCR
- DNA/SNP assay
- DNA/Spectrophotometry
- DNA/Tissue microarray
- Morphology/Standard H&E microscopy
- Morphology/Subcellular localization
- Morphology/Ultrastructure
- Protein/1D/2D gels

- Protein/Antibody microarray
- Protein/Immunohistochemistry
- Protein/Mass Spec
- Protein/Microarray
- Protein/SELDI-TOF Mass Spectrometry[7]
- Protein/Tissue microarray
- Protein/Westerns
- RNA/cDNA Microarray
- RNA/Electrophoresis
- RNA/In situ hybridization
- RNA/Northerns
- RNA/RT-PCR
- RNA/Spectrophotometry
- RNA/Tissue microarray

---

[7] SELDI-TOF is surface-enhanced laser desorption/ionization time-of-flight.

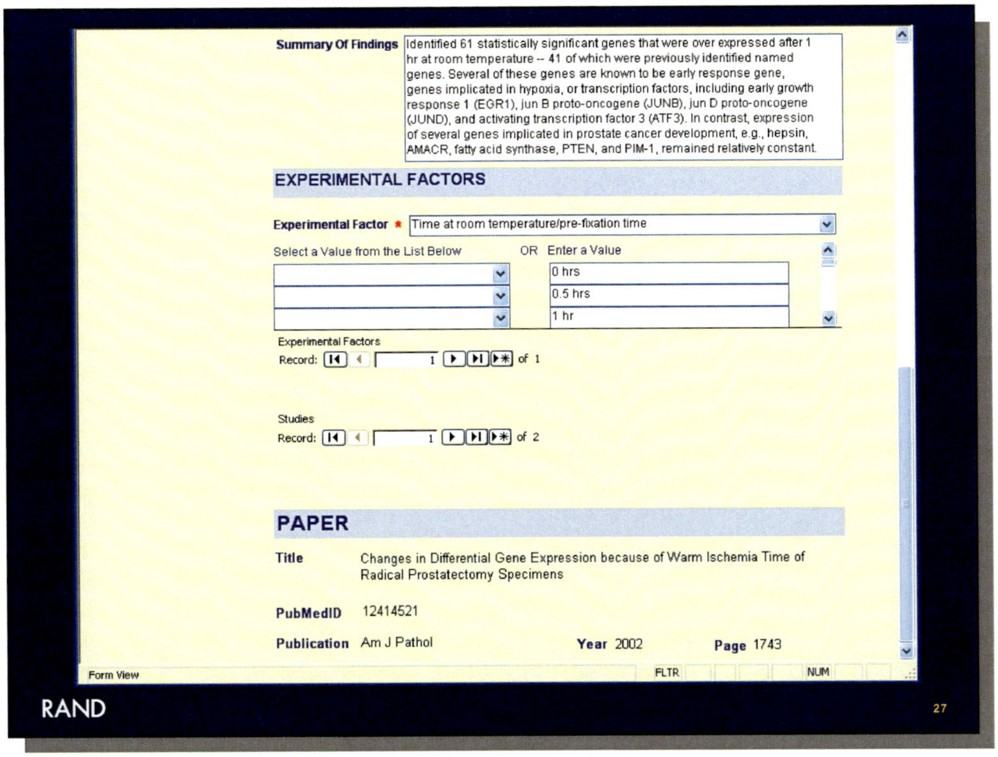

The bottom half of the Studies form contains a free-text box to record a summary of the findings of the study and drop-down menus to record information about the experimental factors. The "Experimental Factors" drop-down menu contains the same choices for the preacquisition and postacquisition variables described earlier for the Excel template with the addition of "RNAase inactivation" and "heterogeneity of specimen aliquots" as postacquisition variables. There is also a choice for "New Factor," which replaces the choice of "Other" on the Excel template, that can be used to record new preacquisition and postacquisition variables that are not already found on the drop-down menu. The experimental factors are tagged as either preacquisition or postacquisition variables in the database even though that classification does not appear on the Studies form to allow for future analysis of the database.

The fields labeled "Select a Value from the List Below" and "Enter a Value" are used to enter more detailed information about the experimental factor being investigated. Once the experimental factor is chosen, only the specific values associated with that experimental factor are displayed in the "Select a Value from the List Below" drop-down menu. Currently, "Type of Fixative" is the only experimental factor that has values available for selection. So if "Type of Fixative" is selected as the experimental factor, a drop-down menu containing choices of different types of fixatives (e.g., ethanol fixation, formalin fixation, OCT, RNAlater,

TRIzol® reagent) is displayed. For experimental factors that do not currently have values listed in the database, the "Enter a Value" boxes allow the entry of free text to enter data. For example, if the experimental factor chosen is "Time at room temperature/pre-fixation time," the times the biospecimens were held at room temperature before they were put into fixative could be recorded in the "Enter a Value" boxes (e.g., 0, 0.5, and 1 hour). It is possible to record multiple experimental factors for a study using the "Experimental Factors Record" navigation tools.

The title of the paper, its PubMed identification number, the journal name, page number, and publication year are displayed at the bottom of the Studies form. It is possible to move between studies within a paper using the "Studies Record" navigation tools.

CHAPTER THREE. LITERATURE-SEARCH STRATEGIES TO IDENTIFY STUDIES ON THE EFFECTS OF PREANALYTICAL VARIABLES

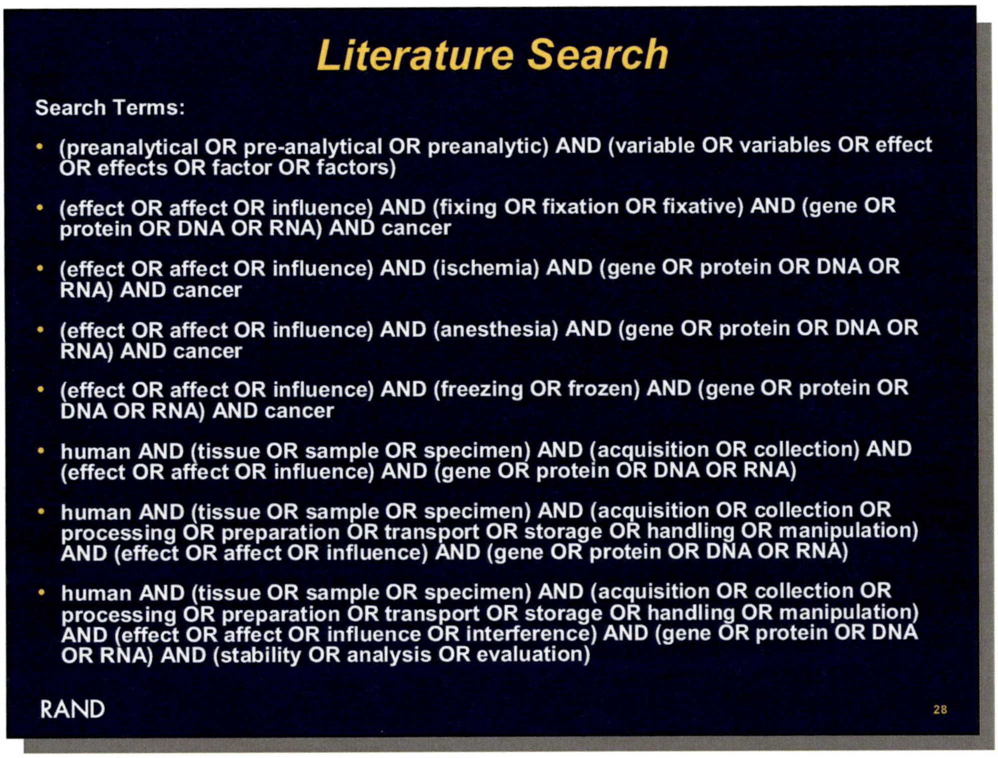

A comprehensive search of the scientific literature was performed to identify studies conducted specifically to determine the effects of preanalytical variables on the quality of biospecimens used to study genetic and proteomic changes in cancer, as well as studies that address methods and technologies for measuring and monitoring changes in biomolecule expression in response to preanalytical variables. To accomplish this, RAND developed a literature-search strategy designed to find studies of interest. Papers were selected to populate the database using several literature-search strategies, including keyword searches, MeSH term searches, and author searches. Each of these search strategies is described in more detail in this chapter.

Keyword searches of PubMed were conducted using a targeted set of search terms to find relevant articles. Searches ranged from very specific, such as the search for *preanalytical variable* and variations thereof and the search using the terms *effect*, *fixation*, *gene*, *protein*, *DNA*, *RNA*, and *cancer* (shown at the top of the slide) to very broad, general searches, such as those using variations of the terms *human*, *specimen*, *acquisition*, *processing*, *storage*, *effect*, *gene*, *protein*, *DNA*, *RNA*, and *analysis* (shown at the bottom of the slide). Other relevant Web sites were also searched, including journals that feature biological methods (e.g., *BioTechniques*, *Cell Preservation Technology* [now *Biopreservation and Biobanking*]). Searches for relevant studies also included the examination of the reference lists from articles already retrieved.

A search of PubMed was performed to identify relevant papers authored by a target list of investigators who are active in the field of biospecimen research. The search was performed using the "Author" field in PubMed for the following:

> (jewell s) OR (grizzle w) OR (LiVolsi V) OR (Hewitt S) OR (Vaught J) OR (Aamodt R) OR (Becich M) OR (Beck J) OR (Buckler A) OR (Figg W) OR (Gunter E) OR (Libutti S) OR (Camphausen K)

The time period specified for the searches covered the past 20 years (i.e., from 1987 through 2007). While many relevant studies were found in papers published more than 10 years ago (i.e., papers published before 1997), it was decided that more recent papers (i.e., papers published between 1997 and 2007) would be of most relevance to the research community and were selected as a place to start to populate the database. Only studies that used human biospecimens were included in the database; studies using biospecimens from other animal sources were not analyzed. Also, only original research articles were included in the database; review articles were not included.

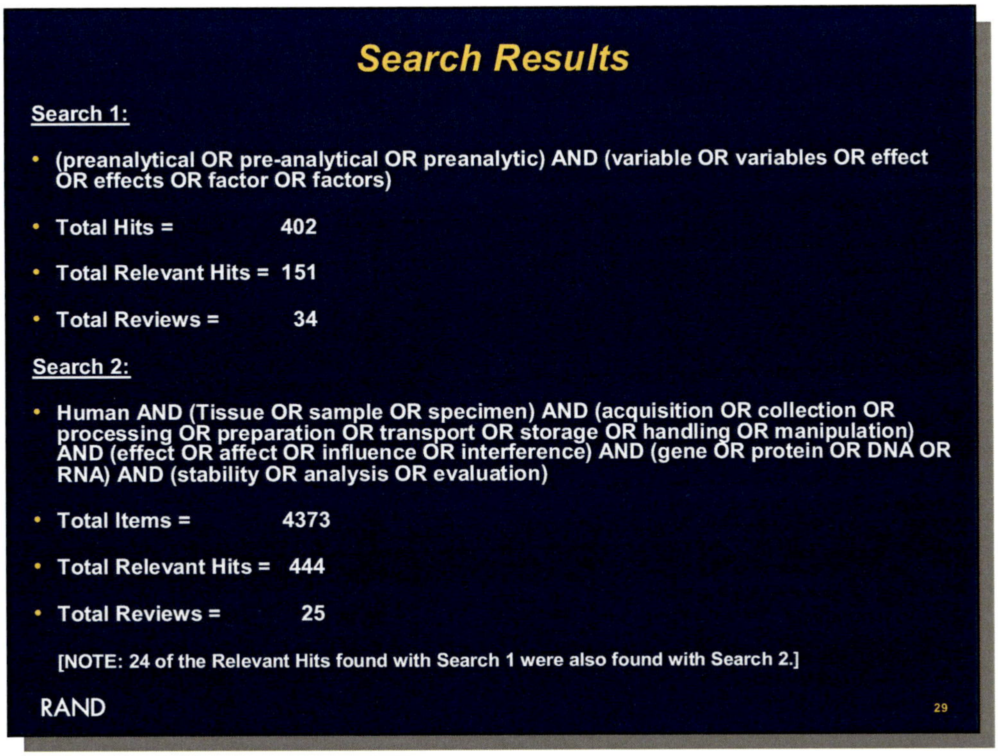

Shown here are search results from two of the keyword searches that were performed in PubMed. Each citation returned was examined for relevance by reviewing the title and abstract (when available). Papers were deemed relevant if they contained studies conducted specifically to determine the effects of preanalytical variables on the quality of biospecimens used to study genetic or proteomic changes in cancer or if they contained studies that addressed methods and technologies for measuring and monitoring changes in biomolecule expression in response to preanalytical variables.

The first search for variations of *preanalytical variable* was fairly specific, yielding 402 total hits, with 151 (or approximately 38 percent) of those hits being selected as relevant. Another 34 hits were for review articles. The second search, using variations of the terms *human*, *specimen*, *acquisition*, *processing*, *storage*, *effect*, *gene*, *protein*, *DNA*, *RNA*, and *analysis*, was much broader in scope and returned 4,373 total hits, with 444 (or approximately 10 percent) of those hits selected as relevant. It is interesting to note that 24 of the relevant hits found with search 1 were also found with search 2.

Each paper selected as relevant to the project was then categorized according to the subject area it covered using the following categorization schema.

Clinical Laboratory Testing and Pathology

I. cells
  a. sperm
  b. buccal cells

II. fluids
  a. blood (e.g., whole blood, serum, plasma, platelets)
    i. coagulation
    ii. chemistry (e.g., pH, electrolytes, gases)
    iii. biochemical markers
      1. cytokines/growth factors
      2. C-reactive protein
      3. hemophilia factors (e.g., factor VIII)
      4. homocysteine/cysteine
      5. insulin
      6. metalloproteinases
      7. parathyroid hormone (PTH)
      8. prostate-specific antigen (PSA)
      9. prothrombin
      10. others
    iv. antidoping (e.g., erythropoietin)
    v. lipids/lipoproteins
    vi. other types of blood testing
  b. urine
  c. fecal samples
  d. saliva
  e. bone marrow
  f. cerebrospinal fluid (CSF)
    i. amyloid beta peptide
  g. amniotic fluid/maternal blood (i.e., whole blood, serum, plasma)
  h. other fluids

III. tissues
  a. brain
  b. breast
  c. heart
  d. liver
  e. other tissues

IV. virology/bacteriology
  a. cytomegalovirus
  b. HIV
  c. hepatitis.

Biomolecule/Technology Platform

I. proteins
   a. microarrays
   b. mass spectroscopy (e.g., SELDI-TOF, matrix-assisted laser desorption/ionization–time of flight [MALDI-TOF], liquid chromatography–mass spectrometry [LC-MS])
   c. immunoassays (e.g., enzyme-linked immunosorbant assay [ELISA], immunohistochemistry, radioimmunoassay)
   d. Western blotting
   e. 2D gel electrophoresis

II. DNA
   a. PCR/real-time PCR
   b. FISH
   c. DNA microarray
   d. CGH
   e. DNA flow/image cytometry

III. mRNA
   a. reverse-transcription/real-time PCR
   b. cDNA microarray
   c. in situ hybridization

IV. morphology
   a. standard H&E
   b. subcellular localization
   c. ultrastructure.

Other Areas of Interest

I. epidemiology

II. biospecimen banking.

Approximately 70 percent of the relevant papers retrieved using the two searches just described dealt with areas classified in the schema as *clinical laboratory testing and pathology* and focused primarily on testing for blood coagulation, blood chemistry, and blood biochemical markers, as well as virology and bacteriology testing. The remaining 30 percent of relevant papers dealt with areas classified in the schema as *biomolecule/technology platform* and focused primarily on protein, DNA, and mRNA.

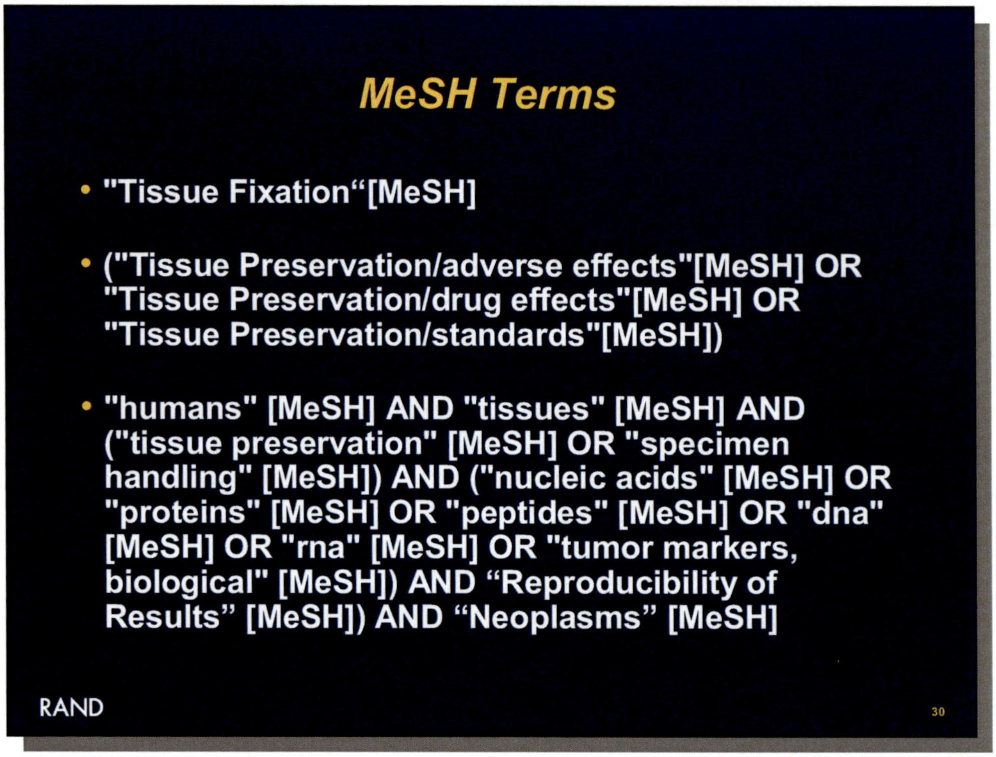

MeSH is the National Library of Medicine's controlled-vocabulary thesaurus used for indexing articles from leading biomedical journals for the PubMed database (NLM, 2008). Each bibliographic reference is associated with a set of MeSH terms that describe the content of the item. Thus, MeSH terms provide "a consistent way to retrieve information that may use different terminology for the same concepts" (NCBI, undated).

Three MeSH term searches were performed to identify additional papers for inclusion in the database. The first search used the MeSH term *tissue fixation*, and the second search used specific MeSH terms under the more general subject heading of *tissue preservation* (i.e., *adverse effects*, *drug effects*, and *standards*). The third search used a more general approach to find relevant papers by combining MeSH terms dealing with *tissue preservation*, *nucleic acids*, *proteins*, and *reproducibility of results*, while focusing on *humans, tissues* and *neoplasms*. The first search yielded 145 hits, the second search yielded 46 hits, and the third search yielded 99 hits. Of all the searches, the search using the MeSH term *tissue fixation* yielded the highest percentage of relevant papers, and 43 of the papers were analyzed and included in the database. In comparison, only three of the papers identified by the second search and two of the papers identified by the third search using MeSH terms were included in the database.

CHAPTER FOUR. DATA ANALYSIS AND STUDY RESULTS

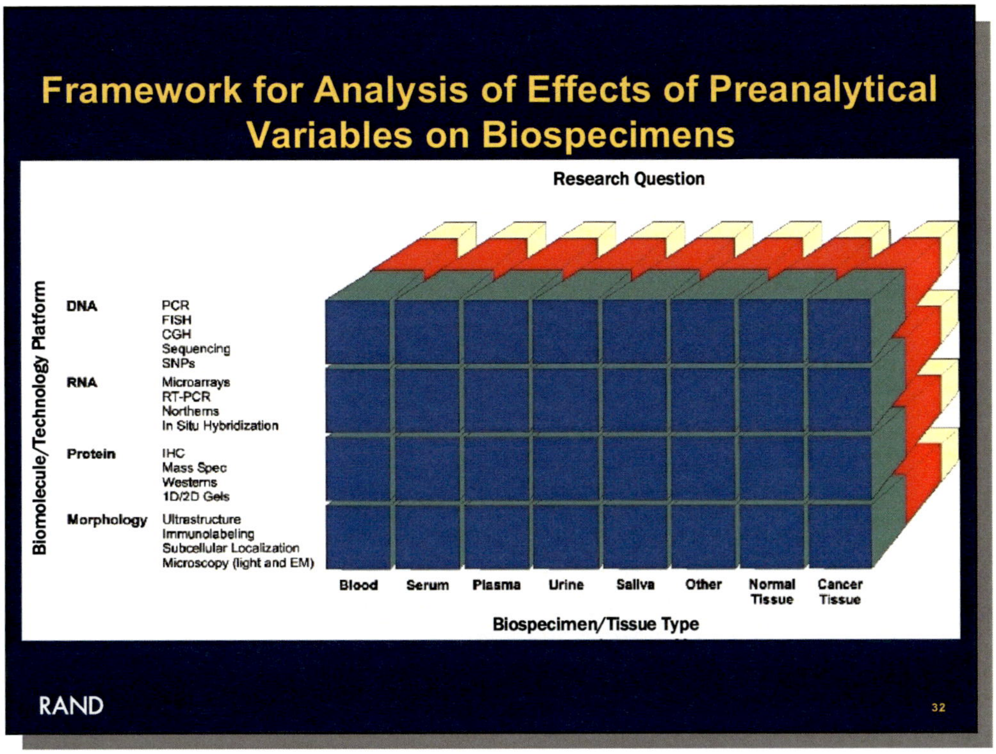

The effects of preanalytical variables on the molecular profile of biospecimens will differ depending on the specimen type (e.g., blood, urine, normal tissue, cancer tissue), the biomolecule being analyzed (e.g., DNA, RNA, protein), the analysis method being used (e.g., Southern blot, PCR, FISH, cDNA microarrays), and the research question being asked. For example, a researcher may want to use cDNA microarray technology to determine the change in expression (i.e., the change in levels of mRNA) of gene X in cancer tissue as compared to normal tissue. Any changes in gene expression due to the acts of acquisition, processing, storage, and distribution of the biospecimen would need to be known in order to distinguish them from changes present in the tissue due to its cancerous state.

One way to conceptualize these preanalytical variables and their potential effects is to array them according to the biospecimen type, the analysis method, and the research question being asked, as shown in the slide (Barker et al., 2005). The three-dimensional array has the biospecimen types along the x-axis, the biomolecule types and associated analysis methods along the y-axis, and the research questions along the z-axis (the blue, red, and off-white colors depict different research questions). This array, developed by OBBR, provides a useful framework for the analysis of the effects of preanalytical variables on biospecimens. By systematically filling in the boxes in the array for each biospecimen type with information about the effects of preanalytical variables on the technology platform used and the research question asked, insight can be gained into the specific impact of different preanalytical variables on the molecular profile of the biospecimen.

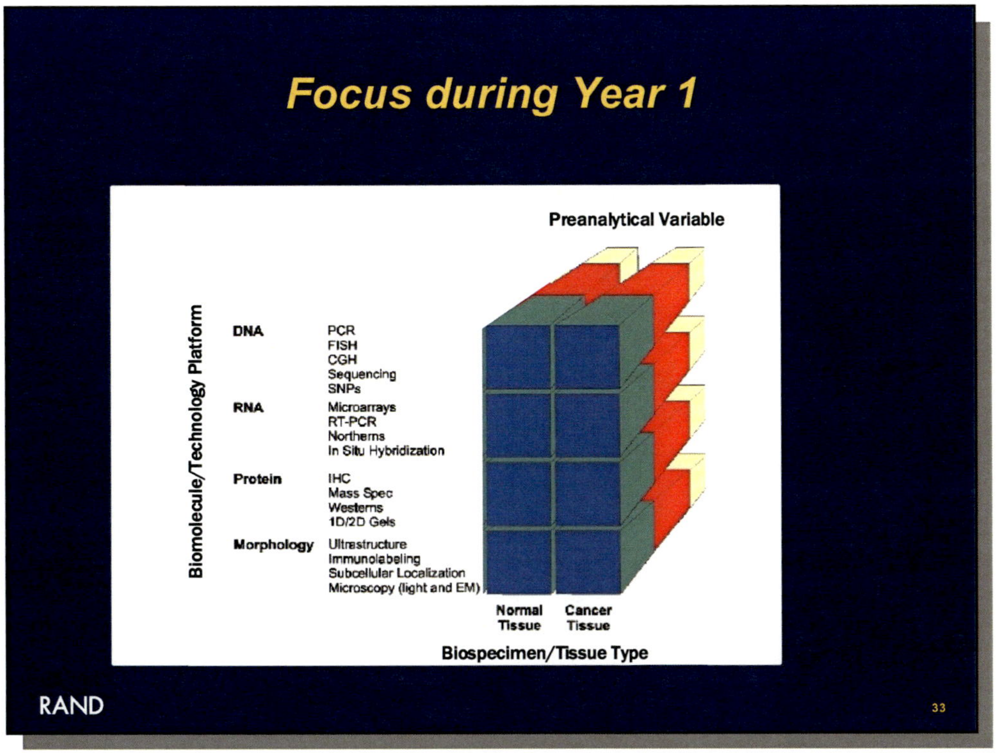

The focus during year 1 of this project was specifically on studies conducted to determine the effects of preanalytical variables on the quality of biospecimens used to study genetic and proteomic changes in cancer. Since studies in the database were limited to those examining cancerous and normal tissue, the only relevant biospecimen/tissue types in the array would be cancerous and normal tissue. In addition, the research question the database is trying to answer is this: How are biospecimens affected by preanalytical variables? This question must be asked for each biomolecule type and technology platform used. Based on the scope of work during year 1 of the project, the framework for analysis of the data in the Biospecimen Research Database could be depicted as a truncated version of the array shown on the previous slide.

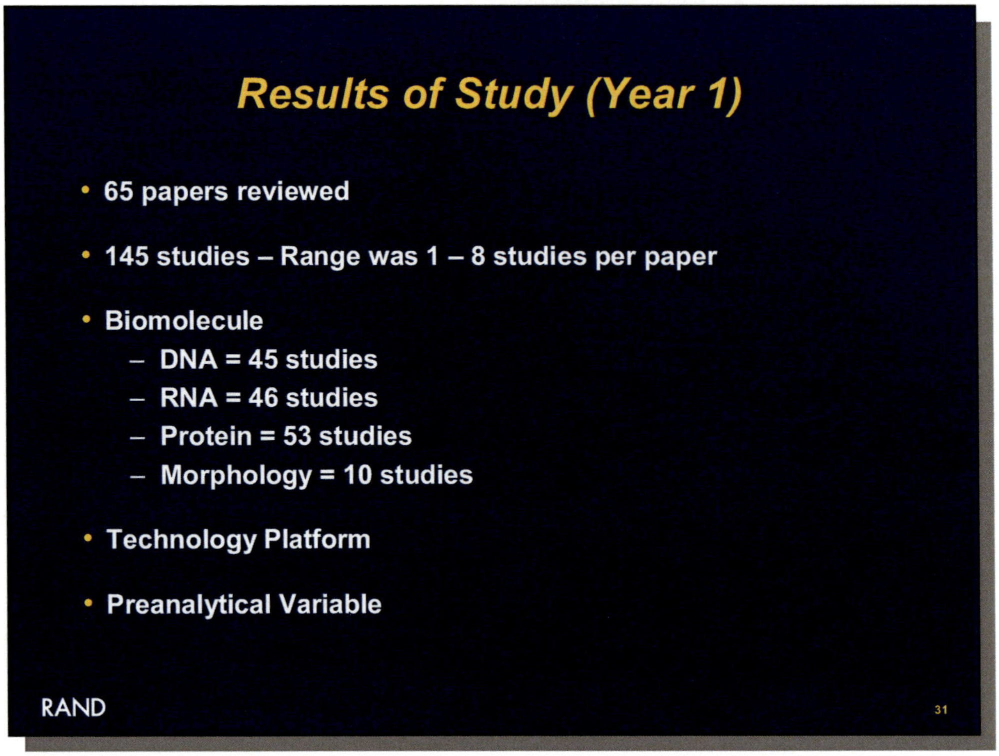

At the time of the briefing to OBBR, 145 studies from 65 papers had been analyzed and entered into the database. The number of studies per paper ranged from one to eight, with most papers containing one, two, or three studies. Of the 145 studies, 45 studies analyzed DNA as the biomolecule, 46 analyzed RNA, 53 analyzed proteins, and 10 analyzed morphology (note that each study may include more than one biomolecule type). The studies used 22 different technology platforms and reported on 15 preanalytical variables. (More detailed information about the technology platforms and preanalytical variables is presented next.) Currently, there are data from 193 studies from 80 papers in the database (references for the 80 papers contained in the Biospecimen Research Database can be found in the appendix).

Technology Platform

Biomolecule	Technology Platform	# of Studies
DNA	Array CGH	5
	CGH	2
	DNA Sequencing	5
	Electrophoresis	8
	FISH	2
	In situ hybridization	1
	PCR	13
	SNP Assay	2
	Tissue Microarray	3
RNA	cDNA Microarray	11
	RT-PCR	24
	Electrophoresis	4
	In situ hybridization	2
	Northerns	4
Protein	SELDI-TOF Mass Spectrometry	5
	Mass Spec	5
	Antibody microarray	2
	Immunohistochemistry	19
	Westerns	8
	Tissue Microarray	3
	1D/2D gels	11
Morphology	Standard H&E microscopy	10

RAND 34

The papers included in the database provided a fairly good representation of the various technology platforms that can be used to study genetic and proteomic changes in cancer. There were 22 different technology platforms used in the studies analyzed for the Biospecimen Research Database. The most commonly used technology platforms were RT-PCR to analyze RNA, immunohistochemistry to analyze proteins, and PCR to analyze DNA. The only technology platforms listed in the database that were not used were tissue microarrays to analyze RNA and subcellular localization and ultrastructure studies to analyze cell morphology.

Preanalytical Variables

Experimental Factor	# of Studies	# of Values
Time at room temperature/ pre-fixation time	16	51
Type of fixative	59	144
Time in fixative	13	36
Biomolecule extraction method	37	77
Storage temperature	8	26
Storage duration	11	44

RAND 35

Within a study, it was possible to have more than one experimental factor (i.e., preanalytical variable), each of which may have several values associated with it. There were 15 different experimental factors identified in the papers analyzed, three of which were preacquisition variables and 12 of which were postacquisition variables. The six most commonly investigated experimental factors were all postacquisition variables: time at room temperature/pre-fixation time, type of fixative, time in fixative, biomolecule extraction method, storage temperature, and storage duration.

Most experimental factors had several associated values. The number of associated values ranged from one to eight, with most experimental factors having two associated values. For example, *time in fixative* typically had several associated values, since each time point in an experiment using a time course would be a new value (e.g., 15 minutes, 30 minutes, 1 hour, 2 hours, 3 hours, 4 hours, 5 hours).

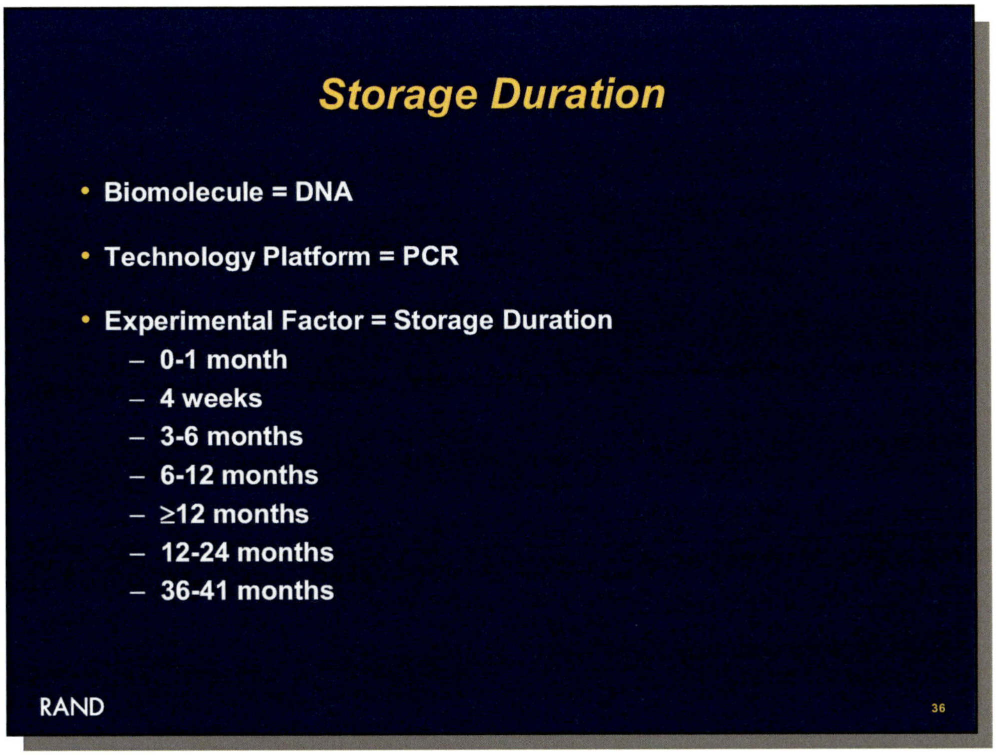

The next step would be to use the information in the Biospecimen Research Database to start to fill in the array just described. Take, for example, studies investigating the effects of differing times in storage (i.e., storage duration) on the ability to amplify DNA from normal tissue and breast cancer biopsies using PCR. The preanalytical variable is *storage duration*, the technology platform is *PCR*, the biomolecule is *DNA*, and the biospecimen/tissue types are *normal tissue* and *cancer tissue*. Figure 4.1 depicts how the information in the database could be used to start filling in the array. The two boxes at the top of the array that are highlighted in yellow correspond to the biospecimen/tissue type and biomolecule/technology platform being analyzed. The preanalytical variable being investigated (i.e., the research question being asked) is the effects of storage duration, shown at the top of the figure.

However, when the data are looked at more closely, it is clear that making comparisons may be difficult. There were 11 studies in the database that examined the effect of storage duration on biospecimens. Depending on the study, storage duration is reported differently. For example, one study reports storing biospecimens for "12 to 24 months," while another study reports that biospecimens were stored for "≥ 12 months." Another example is one study reporting storing biospecimens for "0 to 1 month" and a second study reporting storing biospecimens for 4 weeks. Can these storage times be compared? While it may be possible in this example to compare studies with similar duration times (e.g., 0 to 1 month of storage could be compared to 4 weeks of storage), not all comparisons will be as straightforward. Because of differences in the way in which data are reported in the literature, meta-analyses of the data in the Biospecimen Research Database may be complicated.

Figure 4.1. Framework for Analysis of Effects of Storage Duration on Amplification of DNA from Normal and Cancerous Tissue

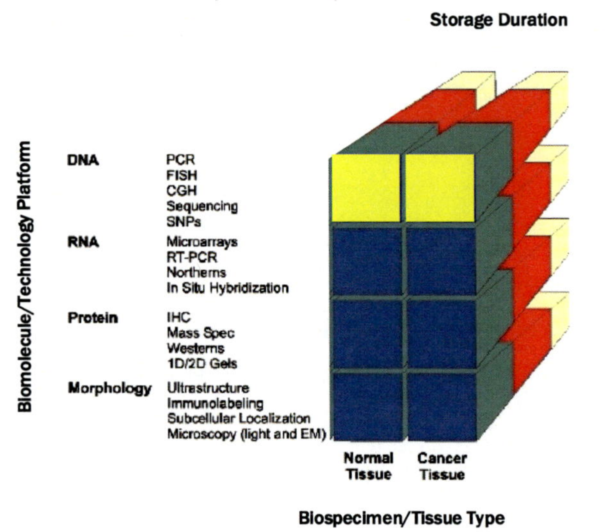

CHAPTER FIVE. CHALLENGES AND NEXT STEPS

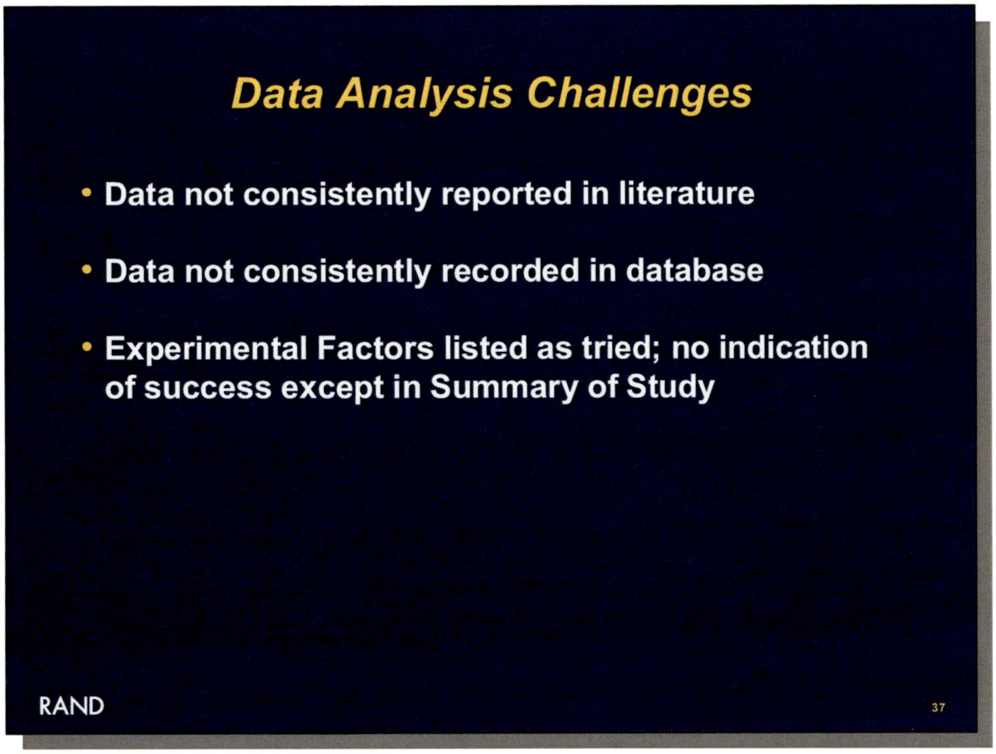

There are some challenges when it comes to analyzing the data in the Biospecimen Research Database. As mentioned in Chapter Four, data on the effects of preanalytical variables on biospecimens are not reported consistently in the literature, a fact that may make comparisons between studies and analyses across studies difficult (i.e., meta-analysis). As the amount of data in the database grows, it may be possible to group studies to make comparisons, but the inconsistencies may make meta-analyses unfeasible. As such, the database may be most useful as a tool to identify gaps in research on the effects of preanalytical variables on biospecimens in which additional studies may be valuable.

Consistency in recording data in the database is also crucial to be able to make comparisons between studies and perform meta-analyses. Drop-down menus with controlled vocabularies were used to help prevent variation from being introduced into the database by the curation process. Limiting or even eliminating the use of free-text boxes to record important findings would also be helpful. Another way in which variation was controlled was by using a second person to review the accuracy of the entries in the database and ensure consistency across data entered by different curators.

Another challenge in analyzing the data is the way in which the effects of preanalytical variables (i.e., the results of the studies) are recorded. Currently, preanalytical variables are selected from a drop-down menu in the data-curation tool, allowing researchers using the Biospecimen Research Database to easily identify which preanalytical variables were investigated in the study. In contrast, the results of the study are recorded in a free-text box (i.e., "Summary of Findings"), making it more difficult to identify what effect, if any, the preanalytical variable had on the biospecimen used, the biomolecule analyzed, or the research question asked. A more systematic way is needed to record and easily identify which preanalytical variables had an effect and what those effects were.

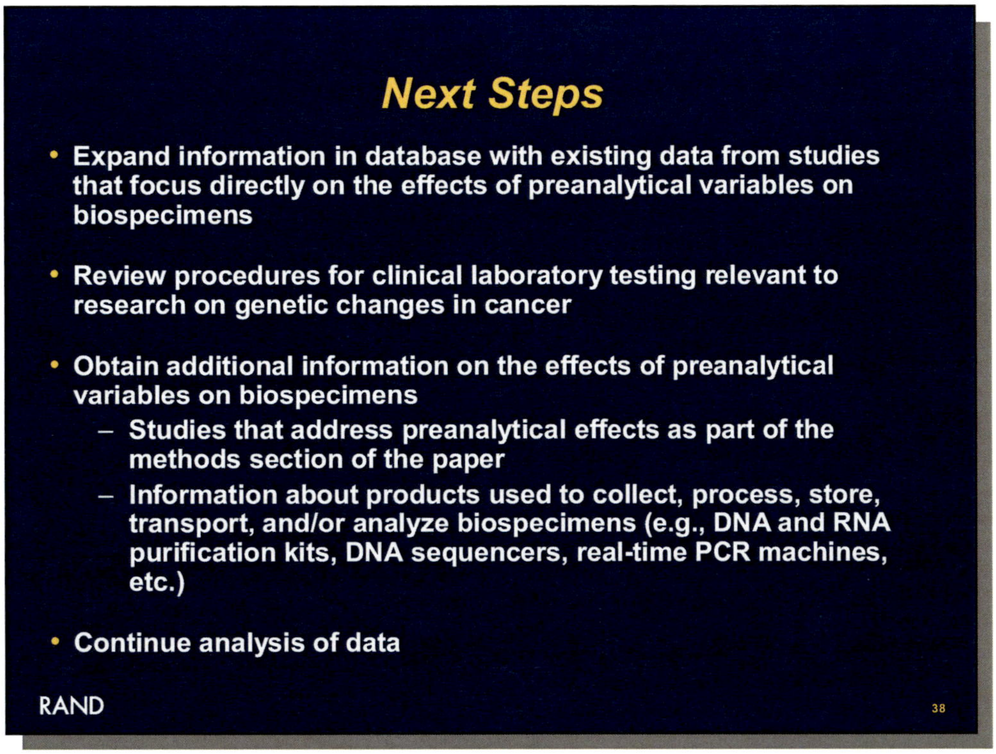

The next steps for the Biospecimen Research Database include expanding the information in the database with data from additional studies that focus directly on the effects of preanalytical variables on biospecimens, as well as adding information from clinical laboratory testing procedures relevant to research on genetic and proteomic changes in cancer (e.g., genetic testing, cytogenetics, molecular pathology). Information may also be obtained from studies that address preanalytical effects as part of the methodology section of the paper. In addition, information may be available from technical-support documents that accompany products used to collect, process, store, transport, or analyze biospecimens (e.g., DNA and RNA purification kits, DNA sequencers, real-time PCR machines). Eventually, it may be feasible to obtain unpublished data on the effects of preanalytical variables on biospecimens from investigators who are active in the field of biospecimen research.

As the database grows, it will be possible to fill in more boxes in the array and to fill each box with sufficient information to be able to start performing analyses of the effects of preanalytical variables on the biospecimens. These data could be used to identify gaps in knowledge about the effects of preanalytical variables and to support the development of guidelines and evidence-based standards for the collection, processing, and storage of biospecimens. The ultimate goal of the database is to provide information to OBBR and the scientific community that will optimize the quality, accessibility, and utility of biospecimens for research purposes.

APPENDIX. REFERENCE LIST FOR PAPERS ANALYZED IN THE BIOSPECIMEN RESEARCH DATABASE

This appendix contains the reference list for the papers that were analyzed in the Biospecimen Research Database.

Abrahamsen, Helene Nortvig, Torben Steiniche, Ebba Nexo, Stephen J. Hamilton-Dutoit, and Boe Sandahl Sorensen, "Towards Quantitative mRNA Analysis in Paraffin-Embedded Tissues Using Real-Time Reverse Transcriptase-Polymerase Chain Reaction: A Methodological Study on Lymph Nodes from Melanoma Patients," *Journal of Molecular Diagnostics*, Vol. 5, No. 1, February 2003, pp. 34–41, PMID: 12552078.

Ahram, Mamoun, Michael J. Flaig, John W. Gillespie, Paul H. Duray, W. Marston Linehan, David K. Ornstein, Shulan Niu, Yingming Zhao, Emanuel F. Petricoin III, and Michael R. Emmert-Buck, "Evaluation of Ethanol-Fixed, Paraffin-Embedded Tissues for Proteomic Applications," *Proteomics*, Vol. 3, No. 4, April 2003, pp. 413–421, PMID: 12687609.

Ahrens, Kim, Raul Braylan, Nidal Almasri, Robin Foss, and Lisa Rimsza, "IgH PCR of Zinc Formalin–Fixed, Paraffin-Embedded Non-Lymphomatous Gastric Samples Produces Artifactual 'Clonal' Bands Not Observed in Paired Tissues Unexposed to Zinc Formalin," *Journal of Molecular Diagnostics*, Vol. 4, No. 3, August 2002, pp. 159–163, PMID: 12169677.

Ananthanarayanan, V., M. R. Pins, R. E. Meyer, and P. H. Gann, "Immunohistochemical Assays in Prostatic Biopsies Processed in Bouin's Fixative," *Journal of Clinical Pathology*, Vol. 58, No. 3, March 2005, pp. 322–324, PMID: 15735170.

Arber, Daniel A., "Effect of Prolonged Formalin Fixation on the Immunohistochemical Reactivity of Breast Markers," *Applied Immunohistochemistry and Molecular Morphology*, Vol. 10, No. 2, June 2002, pp. 183–186, PMID: 12051639.

Beatty, Barbara G., Ronald Bryant, Weichen Wang, Takamaru Ashikaga, Pamela C. Gibson, Gladwyn Leiman, and Donald L. Weaver, "HER-2/neu Detection in Fine-Needle Aspirates of Breast Cancer: Fluorescence In Situ Hybridization and Immunocytochemical Analysis," *American Journal of Clinical Pathology*, Vol. 122, No. 2, August 2004, pp. 246–255, PMID: 15323142.

Becker, K.-F., C. Schott, S. Hipp, V. Metzger, P. Porschewski, R. Beck, J. Nährig, I. Becker, and H. Höfler, "Quantitative Protein Analysis from Formalin-Fixed Tissues: Implications for Translational Clinical Research and Nanoscale Molecular Diagnosis," *Journal of Pathology*, Vol. 211, No. 3, February 2007, pp. 370–378, PMID: 17133373.

Benoy, Ina H., Hilde Elst, Peter Van Dam, Simon Scharpe, Eric Van Marck, Peter B. Vermeulen, and Luc Y. Dirix, "Detection of Circulating Tumour Cells in Blood by Quantitative Real-Time RT-PCR: Effect of Pre-Analytical Time," *Clinical Chemistry and Laboratory Medicine*, Vol. 44, No. 9, 2006, pp. 1082–1087, PMID: 16958599.

Birrell, Geoff W., Jonathan R. Ramsay, Jeffrey J. Tung, and Martin F. Lavin, "Exon Skipping in the ATM Gene in Normal Individuals: The Effect of Blood Sample Storage on RT-PCR Analysis," *Human Mutation*, Vol. 17, No. 1, 2001, pp. 75–76, PMID: 11139252.

Blackhall, Fiona H., Melania Pintilie, Dennis A. Wigle, Igor Jurisica, Ni Liu, Nikolina Radulovich, Michael R. Johnston, Shaf Keshavjee, and Ming-Sound Tsao, "Stability and Heterogeneity of Expression Profiles in Lung Cancer Specimens Harvested Following Surgical Resection," *Neoplasia*, Vol. 6, No. 6, November–December 2004, pp. 761–767, PMID: 15720802.

Bonin, S., F. Petrera, J. Rosai, and G. Stanta, "DNA and RNA Obtained from Bouin's Fixed Tissues," *Journal of Clinical Pathology*, Vol. 58, No. 3, March 2005, pp. 313–316, PMID: 15735167.

Breit, S., M. Nees, U. Schaefer, M. Pfoersich, C. Hagemeier, M. Muckenthaler, and A. E. Kulozik, "Impact of Pre-Analytical Handling on Bone Marrow mRNA Gene Expression," *British Journal of Haematology*, Vol. 126, No. 2, July 2004, pp. 231–243, PMID: 15238145.

Chan, K. C. Allen, Sze-Wan Yeung, Wing-Bong Lui, Timothy H. Rainer, and Y. M. Dennis Lo, "Effects of Preanalytical Factors on the Molecular Size of Cell-Free DNA in Blood," *Clinical Chemistry*, Vol. 51, No. 4, April 2005, pp. 781–784, PMID: 15708950.

Chu, Wei-Sing, Bungo Furusato, Kondi Wong, Isabell A. Sesterhenn, Fathollah K. Mostofi, Min Qi Wei, Zhenqing Zhu, Susan L. Abbondanzo, and Qi Liang, "Ultrasound-Accelerated Formalin Fixation of Tissue Improves Morphology, Antigen and mRNA Preservation," *Modern Pathology*, Vol. 18, No. 6, June 2005, pp. 850–863, PMID: 15605077.

Chu, Wei-Sing, Qi Liang, Jilan Liu, Min Qi Wei, Mary Winters, Lance Liotta, Glenn Sandberg, and Maokai Gong, "A Nondestructive Molecule Extraction Method Allowing Morphological and Molecular Analyses Using a Single Tissue Section," *Laboratory Investigation*, Vol. 85, No. 11, November 2005, pp. 1416–1428, PMID: 16127423.

Chu, Wei-Sing, Qi Liang, Yao Tang, Randy King, Kondi Wong, Maokai Gong, Minqi Wei, Jilan Liu, Shaw-Huey Feng, Shyh-Ching Lo, Jo-Ann Andriko, and Marshall Orr, "Ultrasound-Accelerated Tissue Fixation/Processing Achieves Superior Morphology and Macromolecule Integrity with Storage Stability," *Journal of Histochemistry and Cytochemistry*, Vol. 54, No. 5, May 2006, pp. 503–513, PMID: 16314441.

Chung, J. Y., T. Braunschweig, and S. M. Hewitt, "Optimization of Recovery of RNA from Formalin-Fixed, Paraffin-Embedded Tissue," *Diagnostic Molecular Pathology*, Vol. 15, No. 4, December 2006, pp. 229–236, PMID: 17122651.

Coura, R., J. C. Prolla, L. Meurer, and P. Ashton-Prolla, "An Alternative Protocol for DNA Extraction from Formalin Fixed and Paraffin Wax Embedded Tissue," *Journal of Clinical Pathology*, Vol. 58, No. 8, August 2005, pp. 894–895, PMID: 16049299.

Dash, Atreya, Ira P. Maine, Sooryanarayana Varambally, Ronglai Shen, Arul M. Chinnaiyan, and Mark A. Rubin, "Changes in Differential Gene Expression Because of Warm Ischemia Time of Radical Prostatectomy Specimens," *American Journal of Pathology*, Vol. 161, No. 5, November 2002, pp. 1743–1748, PMID: 12414521.

De Marzo, A. M., H. H. Fedor, W. R. Gage, and M. A. Rubin, "Inadequate Formalin Fixation Decreases Reliability of p27 Immunohistochemical Staining: Probing Optimal Fixation Time Using High-Density Tissue Microarrays," *Human Pathology*, Vol. 33, No. 7, July 2002, pp. 756–760, PMID: 12196928.

Derecskei, Katalin, Judit Moldvay, Krisztina Bogos, and József Tímár, "Protocol Modifications Influence the Result of EGF Receptor

Immunodetection by EGFR pharmDx™ in Paraffin-Embedded Cancer Tissues," *Pathology and Oncology Research*, Vol. 12, No. 4, 2006, pp. 243–246, PMID: 17189989.

Djordjevic, V., M. Stankovic, A. Nikolic, N. Antonijevic, L. J. Rakicevic, A. Divac, and M. Radojkovic, "PCR Amplification on Whole Blood Samples Treated with Different Commonly Used Anticoagulants," *Journal of Pediatric Hematology/Oncology*, Vol. 23, No. 6, September 2006, pp. 517–521, PMID: 16849283.

Emerson, Lyska L., Sheryl R. Tripp, Bradley C. Baird, Lester J. Layfield, and Ralph L. Rohr, "A Comparison of Immunohistochemical Stain Quality in Conventional and Rapid Microwave Processed Tissues," *American Journal of Clinical Pathology*, Vol. 125, No. 2, February 2006, pp. 176–183, PMID: 16393680.

Ericsson, Christer, Inti Peredo, and Monica Nister, "Optimized Protein Extraction from Cryopreserved Brain Tissue Samples," *Acta Oncologica*, Vol. 46, No. 1, 2007, pp. 10–20, PMID: 17438701.

Fergenbaum, Jennifer H., Montserrat Garcia-Closas, Stephen M. Hewitt, Jolanta Lissowska, Lori C. Sakoda, and Mark E. Sherman, "Loss of Antigenicity in Stored Sections of Breast Cancer Tissue Microarrays," *Cancer Epidemiology, Biomarkers and Prevention*, Vol. 13, No. 4, April 2004, pp. 667–672, PMID: 15066936.

Finkelstein, Sydney D., Rajiv Dhir, Mordechai Rabinovitz, Michelle Bischeglia, Patrick A. Swalsky, Petrina DeFlavia, Jeffrey Woods, Anke Bakker, and Michael Becich, "Cold-Temperature Plastic Resin Embedding of Liver for DNA- and RNA-Based Genotyping," *Journal of Molecular Diagnostics*, Vol. 1, No. 1, November 1999, pp. 17–22, PMID: 11272904.

Florell, Scott R., Cheryl M. Coffin, Joseph A. Holden, James W. Zimmermann, John W. Gerwels, Bradley K. Summers, David A. Jones, and Sancy A. Leachman, "Preservation of RNA for Functional Genomic Studies: A Multidisciplinary Tumor Bank Protocol," *Modern Pathology*, Vol. 14, No. 2, February 2001, pp. 116–128, PMID: 11235903.

García-Closas, Montserrat, Kathleen M. Egan, Jeannine Abruzzo, Polly A. Newcomb, Linda Titus-Ernstoff, Tracie Franklin, Patrick K. Bender, Jeanne C. Beck, Loïc Le Marchand, Annette Lum, Michael Alavanja, Richard B. Hayes, Joni Rutter, Kenneth Buetow, Louise A. Brinton, and Nathaniel Rothman, "Collection of Genomic DNA from Adults in Epidemiological Studies by Buccal Cytobrush and Mouthwash,"

Cancer Epidemiology, Biomarkers and Prevention, Vol 10, No. 6, June 2001, pp. 687–696, PMID: 11401920.

Gillespie, John W., Carolyn J. M. Best, Verena E. Bichsel, Kristina A. Cole, Susan F. Greenhut, Stephen M. Hewitt, Mamoun Ahram, Yvonne B. Gathright, Maria J. Merino, Robert L. Strausberg, Jonathan I. Epstein, Stanley R. Hamilton, Gallya Gannot, Galina V. Baibakova, Valerie S. Calvert, Michael J. Flaig, Rodrigo F. Chuaqui, Judi C. Herring, John Pfeifer, Emmanuel F. Petricoin, W. Marston Linehan, Paul H. Duray, G. Steven Bova, and Michael R. Emmert-Buck, "Evaluation of Non-Formalin Tissue Fixation for Molecular Profiling Studies," *American Journal of Pathology*, Vol. 160, No. 2, February 2002, pp. 449–457, PMID: 11839565.

Gjerdrum, L. M., H. N. Abrahamsen, B. Villegas, B. S. Sorensen, H. Schmidt, and S. J. Hamilton-Dutoit, "The Influence of Immunohistochemistry on mRNA Recovery from Microdissected Frozen and Formalin-Fixed, Paraffin-Embedded Sections," *Diagnostic Molecular Pathology*, Vol. 13, No. 4, December 2004, pp. 224–233, PMID: 15538113.

Gloghini, Annunziata, Barbara Canal, Ulf Klein, Luigino Dal Maso, Tiziana Perin, Riccardo Dalla-Favera, and Antonino Carbone, "RT-PCR Analysis of RNA Extracted from Bouin-Fixed and Paraffin-Embedded Lymphoid Tissues," *Journal of Molecular Diagnostics*, Vol. 6, No. 4, November 2004, pp. 290–296, PMID: 15507667.

Goldmann, Torsten, Daniel Drömann, Marouane Marzouki, Udo Schimmel, Karsten Debel, Detlev Branscheid, Tobias Zeiser, Jan Rupp, Johannes Gerdes, Peter Zabel, and Ekkehard Vollmer, "Tissue Microarrays from HOPE-Fixed Specimens Allow for Enhanced High Throughput Molecular Analyses in Paraffin-Embedded Material," *Pathology: Research and Practice*, Vol. 201, Nos. 8–9, 2005, pp. 599–602, PMID: 16259114.

Hood, Brian L., Marlene M. Darfler, Thomas G. Guiel, Bungo Furusato, David A. Lucas, Bradley R. Ringeisen, Isabell A. Sesterhenn, Thomas P. Conrads, Timothy D. Veenstra, and David B. Krizman, "Proteomic Analysis of Formalin-Fixed Prostate Cancer Tissue," *Molecular and Cellular Proteomics*, Vol. 4, No. 11, November 2005, pp. 1741–1753, PMID: 16091476.

Hu, S. P., J. S. Yang, M. Y. Wu, Z. Y. Shen, K. H. Zhang, J. W. Liu, and B. Guan, "Effect of One-Step 100% Ethanol Fixation and Modified Manual Microdissection on High-Quality RNA Recovery from

Esophageal Carcinoma Specimen," *Diseases of the Esophagus*, Vol. 18, No. 3, 2005, pp. 190–198, PMID: 16045582.

Huang, J., R. Qi, J. Quackenbush, E. Dauway, E. Lazaridis, and T. Yeatman, "Effects of Ischemia on Gene Expression," *Journal of Surgical Research*, Vol. 99, No. 2, August 2001, pp. 222–227, PMID: 11469890.

Huang, Q., P. G. Sacks, J. Mo, S. A. McCormick, C. E. Iacob, L. Guo, S. Schaefer, and S. P. Schantz, "A Simple Method for Fixation and Microdissection of Frozen Fresh Tissue Sections for Molecular Cytogenetic Analysis of Cancers," *Biotechnic and Histochemistry*, Vol. 80, Nos. 3–4, May–August 2005, pp. 147–156, PMID: 16298900.

Hummon, Amanda B., Sharlene R. Lim, Michael J. Difilippantonio, and Thomas Ried, "Isolation and Solubilization of Proteins After TRIzol® Extraction of RNA and DNA from Patient Material Following Prolonged Storage," *BioTechniques*, Vol. 42, No. 4, April 2007, pp. 467–470, 472, PMID: 17489233.

Isaksson, Helena S., and Torbjörn K. Nilsson, "Preanalytical Aspects of Quantitative TaqMan Real-Time RT-PCR: Applications for TF and VEGF mRNA Quantification," *Clinical Biochemistry*, Vol. 39, No. 4, April 2006, pp. 373–377, PMID: 16546153.

Jewell, Scott D., Mythily Srinivasan, Linda M. McCart, Nita Williams, William H. Grizzle, Virginia LiVolsi, Greg MacLennan, Daniel D. Sedmak, "Analysis of the Molecular Quality of Human Tissues: An Experience from the Cooperative Human Tissue Network," *American Journal of Clinical Pathology*, Vol. 118, No. 5, November 2002, pp. 733–741, PMID: 12428794.

Jin, L., J. Majerus, A. Oliveira, C. Y. Inwards, A. G. Nascimento, L. J. Burgart, and R. V. Lloyd, "Detection of Fusion Gene Transcripts in Fresh-Frozen and Formalin-Fixed Paraffin-Embedded Tissue Sections of Soft-Tissue Sarcomas After Laser Capture Microdissection and rt-PCR," *Diagnostic Molecular Pathology*, Vol. 12, No. 4, December 2003, pp. 224–230, PMID: 14639108.

Koch, I., J. Slotta-Huspenina, R. Hollweck, N. Anastasov, H. Hofler, L. Quintanilla-Martinez, and F. Fend, "Real-Time Quantitative RT-PCR Shows Variable, Assay-Dependent Sensitivity to Formalin Fixation: Implications for Direct Comparison of Transcript Levels in Paraffin-Embedded Tissues," *Diagnostic Molecular Pathology*, Vol. 15, No. 3, September 2006, pp. 149–156, PMID: 16932070.

Lee, H., A. G. Douglas-Jones, J. M. Morgan, and B. Jasani, "The Effect of Fixation and Processing on the Sensitivity of Oestrogen Receptor Assay by Immunohistochemistry in Breast Carcinoma," *Journal of Clinical Pathology*, Vol. 55, No. 3, March 2002, pp. 236–238, PMID: 11896082.

Lin, Daniel W., Lisa M. Coleman, Sarah Hawley, Ruth Dumpit, David Gifford, Philip Kezele, Hau Hung, Beatrice S. Knudsen, Alan R. Kristal, and Peter S. Nelson, "Influence of Surgical Manipulation on Prostate Gene Expression: Implications for Molecular Correlates of Treatment Effects and Disease Prognosis," *Journal of Clinical Oncology*, Vol. 24, No. 23, August 10, 2006, pp. 3763–3770, PMID: 16822846.

Lips, Esther H., Jan Willem F. Dierssen, Ronald van Eijk, Jan Oosting, Paul H. C. Eilers, Rob A. E. M. Tollenaar, Eelco J. de Graaf, Ruben van't Slot, Cisca Wijmenga, Hans Morreau, and Tom van Wezel, "Reliable High-Throughput Genotyping and Loss-of-Heterozygosity Detection in Formalin-Fixed, Paraffin-Embedded Tumors Using Single Nucleotide Polymorphism Arrays," *Cancer Research*, Vol. 65, No. 22, November 15, 2005, pp. 10188–10191, PMID: 16288005.

Little, Suzanne E., Raisa Vuononvirta, Jorge S. Reis-Filho, Rachael Nahajan, Marjan Iravani, Kerry Fenwick, Alan Mackay, Alan Ashworth, Kathy Pritchard-Jones, and Chris Jones, "Array CGH Using Whole Genome Amplification of Fresh-Frozen and Formalin-Fixed, Paraffin-Embedded Tumor DNA," *Genomics*, Vol. 87, No. 2, February 2006, pp. 298–306, PMID: 16271290.

Macabeo-Ong, Maricris, David G. Ginzinger, Nusi Dekker, Alex McMillan, Joseph A. Regezi, David T. W. Wong, and Richard C. K. Jordan, "Effect of Duration of Fixation on Quantitative Reverse Transcription Polymerase Chain Reaction Analyses," *Modern Pathology*, Vol. 15, No. 9, September 2002, pp. 979–987, PMID: 12218216.

Mato, S., and A. Pazos, "Influence of Age, Postmortem Delay and Freezing Storage Period on Cannabinoid Receptor Density and Functionality in Human Brain," *Neuropharmacology*, Vol. 46, No. 5, April 2004, pp. 716–726, PMID: 14996549.

Mehrian Shai, Ruty, Juergen K. V. Reichardt, Hsu Ya-Hsuan, Thomas J. Kremen, Linda M. Liau, Timothy F. Cloughesy, Paul S. Mischel, and Stanley F. Nelson, "Robustness of Gene Expression Profiling in Glioma Specimen Samplings and Derived Cell Lines," *Molecular Brain Research*, Vol. 136, Nos. 1–2, May 20, 2005, pp. 99–103, PMID: 15893592.

Micke, Patrick, Mitsuhiro Ohshima, Simin Tahmasebpoor, Zhi-Ping Ren, Arne Östman, Fredrik Pontén, and Johan Botling, "Biobanking of Fresh Frozen Tissue: RNA Is Stable in Nonfixed Surgical Specimens," *Laboratory Investigation*, Vol. 86, No. 2, February 2006, pp. 202–211, PMID: 16402036.

Miething, Franziska, Sandra Hering, Bärbel Hanschke, and Jan Dressler, "Effect of Fixation to the Degradation of Nuclear and Mitochondrial DNA in Different Tissues," *Journal of Histochemistry and Cytochemistry*, Vol. 54, No. 3, March 2006, pp. 371–374, PMID: 16260588.

Morrison, Carl, Jeff Palatini, Judy Riggenbach, Michael Radmacher, and Pierluigi Porcu, "Fine-Needle Aspiration Biopsy of Non-Hodgkin Lymphoma for Use in Expression Microarray Analysis," *Cancer*, Vol. 108, No. 5, October 25, 2006, pp. 311–318, PMID: 16944538.

Murrell-Bussell, Sarah, Dianne Nguyen, Wendy D. Schober, Jeffrey Scott, Joe Leigh Simpson, Sherman Elias, Farideh Z. Bischoff, and Dorothy E. Lewis, "Optimized Fixation and Storage Conditions for FISH Analysis of Single-Cell Suspensions," *Journal of Histochemistry and Cytochemistry*, Vol. 46, No. 8, August 1998, pp. 971–974, PMID: 9671447.

Mutter, George L., David Zahrieh, Chunmei Liu, Donna Neuberg, David Finkelstein, Heather E. Baker, and Janet A. Warrington, "Comparison of Frozen and RNALater Solid Tissue Storage Methods for Use in RNA Expression Microarrays," *BMC Genomics*, Vol. 5, No. 1, November 10, 2004, p. 88, PMID: 15537428.

Nadji, M., M. Nassiri, V. Vincek, R. Kanhoush, and A. R. Morales, "Immunohistochemistry of Tissue Prepared by a Molecular-Friendly Fixation and Processing System," *Applied Immunohistochemistry and Molecular Morphology*, Vol. 13, No. 3, September 2005, pp. 277–282, PMID: 16082256.

Narayanan, S., M. R. O'Donovan, and S. J. Duthie, "Lysis of Whole Blood In Vitro Causes DNA Strand Breaks in Human Lymphocytes," *Mutagenesis*, Vol. 16, No. 6, November 2001, pp. 455–459, PMID: 11682634.

Ohashi, Yoko, Kim E. Creek, Lucia Pirisi, Ram Kalus, and S. Robert Young, "RNA Degradation in Human Breast Tissue After Surgical Removal: A Time-Course Study," *Experimental and Molecular Pathology*, Vol. 77, No. 2, October 2004, pp. 98–103, PMID: 15351232.

Palmer-Toy, Darryl Erik, Bryan Krastins, David A. Sarracino, Joseph B. Nadol Jr., and Saumil N. Merchant, "Efficient Method for the

Proteomic Analysis of Fixed and Embedded Tissues," *Journal of Proteome Research*, Vol. 4, No. 6, November–December 2005, pp. 2404–2411, PMID: 16335994.

Páska, Csilla, Krisztina Bögi, László Szilák, Annamária Tokés, Erzsébet Szabó, István Sziller, János Rigó, Gábor Sobel, István Szabó, Pál Kaposi-Novák, András Kiss, and Zsuzsa Schaff, "Effect of Formalin, Acetone, and RNAlater Fixatives on Tissue Preservation and Different Size Amplicons by Real-Time PCR from Paraffin-Embedded Tissue," *Diagnostic Molecular Pathology*, Vol. 13, No. 4, December 2004, pp. 234–240, PMID: 15538114.

Perlmutter, Mark A., Carolyn J. M. Best, John W. Gillespie, Yvonne Gathright, Sergio González, Alfredo Velasco, W. Marston Linehan, Michael R. Emmert-Buck, and Rodrigo F. Chuaqui, "Comparison of Snap Freezing Versus Ethanol Fixation for Gene Expression Profiling of Tissue Specimens," *Journal of Molecular Diagnostics*, Vol. 6, No. 4, November 2004, pp. 371–377, PMID: 15507677.

Petersen, B. L., M. C. Sørensen, S. Pedersen, and M. Rasmussen, "Fluorescence In Situ Hybridization on Formalin-Fixed and Paraffin-Embedded Tissue: Optimizing the Method," *Applied Immunohistochemistry and Molecular Morphology*, Vol. 12, No. 3, September 2004, pp. 259–265, PMID: 15551741.

Rai, Alex J., Craig A. Gelfand, Bruce C. Haywood, David J. Warunek, Jizu Yi, Mark D. Schuchard, Richard J. Mehigh, Steven L. Cockrill, Graham B. I. Scott, Harald Tammen, Peter Schulz-Knappe, David W. Speicher, Frank Vitzthum, Brian B. Haab, Gerard Siest, and Daniel W. Chan, "HUPO Plasma Proteome Project Specimen Collection and Handling: Towards the Standardization of Parameters for Plasma Proteome Samples," *Proteomics*, Vol. 5, No. 13, August 2005, pp. 3262–3277, PMID: 16052621.

Rivero, Elena R. C., Adriana C. Neves, Maria G. Silva-Valenzuela, Suzana O. M. Sousa, and Fabio D. Nunes, "Simple Salting-Out Method for DNA Extraction from Formalin-Fixed, Paraffin-Embedded Tissues," *Pathology: Research and Practice*, Vol. 202, No. 7, 2006, pp. 523–529, PMID: 16723190.

Sato, Y., R. Sugie, B. Tsuchiya, T. Kameya, M. Natori, and K. Mukai, "Comparison of the DNA Extraction Methods for Polymerase Chain Reaction Amplification from Formalin-Fixed and Paraffin-Embedded Tissues," *Diagnostic Molecular Pathology*, Vol. 10, No. 4, December 2001, pp. 265–271, PMID: 11763318.

Schoch, Robert, Jurij Pitako, Philippe Schafhausen, Stefan Jenisch, Torsten Haferlach, Michael Kneba, and Meinolf Suttorp, "Semiquantitative Reverse Transcription Polymerase Chain Reaction Analysis for Detection of bcr/abl Rearrangement Using RNA Extracts from Bone Marrow Aspirates Compared with Glass Slide Smears After 0, 2 and 4 D of Storage," *British Journal of Haematology*, Vol. 115, No. 3, December 2001, pp. 583–587, PMID: 11736939.

Schubert, Elizabeth L., Li Hsu, Laura A. Cousens, Jeri Glogovac, Steve Self, Brian J. Reid, Peter S. Rabinovitch, and Peggy L. Porter, "Single Nucleotide Polymorphism Array Analysis of Flow-Sorted Epithelial Cells from Frozen Versus Fixed Tissues for Whole Genome Analysis of Allelic Loss in Breast Cancer," *American Journal of Pathology*, Vol. 160, No. 1, January 2002, pp. 73–79, PMID: 11786401.

Selvarajan, Sathiyamoorthy, Boon-Huat Bay, Andrew Choo, Khoon-Leong Chuah, Christina Rudduck Sivaswaren, Sim-Leng Tien, Chow-Yin Wong, and Puay-Hoon Tan, "Effect of Fixation Period on HER2/neu Gene Amplification Detected by Fluorescence In Situ Hybridization in Invasive Breast Carcinoma," *Journal of Histochemistry and Cytochemistry*, Vol. 50, No. 12, December 2002, pp. 1693–1696; erratum in *Journal of Histochemistry and Cytochemistry*, Vol. 51, No. 2, February 2003, p. 267, PMID: 12486093.

Shi, Shan-Rong, Ram Datar, Cheng Liu, Lin Wu, Zina Zhang, Richard J. Cote, and Clive R. Taylor, "DNA Extraction from Archival Formalin-Fixed, Paraffin-Embedded Tissues: Heat-Induced Retrieval in Alkaline Solution," *Histochemistry and Cell Biology*, Vol. 122, No. 3, September 2004, pp. 211–218, PMID: 15322858.

Sigurdson, Alice J., Mina Ha, Mark Cosentino, Tracie Franklin, Kashif A. Haque, Ying Qi, Cynthia Glaser, Yvonne Reid, Jim B. Vaught, and Andrew W. Bergen, "Long-Term Storage and Recovery of Buccal Cell DNA from Treated Cards," *Cancer Epidemiology, Biomarkers and Prevention*, Vol. 15, No. 2, February 2006, pp. 385–388, PMID: 16492933.

Sozzi, Gabriella, Luca Roz, Davide Conte, Luigi Mariani, Francesca Andriani, Paolo Verderio, and Ugo Pastorino, "Effects of Prolonged Storage of Whole Plasma or Isolated Plasma DNA on the Results of Circulating DNA Quantification Assays," *Journal of the National Cancer Institute*, Vol. 97, No. 24, December 21, 2005, pp. 1848–1850, PMID: 16368947.

Specht, Katja, Thomas Richter, Ulrike Muller, Axel Walch, Martin Werner, and Heinz Höfler, "Quantitative Gene Expression Analysis in

Microdissected Archival Formalin-Fixed and Paraffin-Embedded Tumor Tissue," *American Journal of Pathology*, Vol. 158, No. 2, February 2001, pp. 419–429, PMID: 11159180.

Spruessel, Annika, Garnet Steimann, Mira Jung, Sung A. Lee, Theresa Carr, Anne-Kristin Fentz, Joerg Spangenberg, Carsten Zornig, Hartmut H. Juhl, and Kerstin A. David, "Tissue Ischemia Time Affects Gene and Protein Expression Patterns Within Minutes Following Surgical Tumor Excision," *BioTechniques*, Vol. 36, No. 6, June 2004, pp. 1030–1037, PMID: 15211754.

Thompson, Ella R., Shane C. Herbert, Susan M. Forrest, and Ian G. Campbell, "Whole Genome SNP Arrays Using DNA Derived from Formalin-Fixed, Paraffin-Embedded Ovarian Tumor Tissue," *Human Mutation*, Vol. 26, No. 4, October 2005, pp. 384–389, PMID: 16116623.

Titford, Michael E., and Marcelo G. Horenstein, "Histomorphologic Assessment of Formalin Substitute Fixatives for Diagnostic Surgical Pathology," *Archives of Pathology and Laboratory Medicine*, Vol. 129, No. 4, April 2005, pp. 502–506, PMID: 15794674.

Uhlig, U., S. Uhlig, D. Branscheid, P. Zabel, E. Vollmer, and T. Goldmann, "HOPE Technique Enables Western Blot Analysis from Paraffin-Embedded Tissues," *Pathology: Research and Practice*, Vol. 200, No. 6, 2004, pp. 469–472, PMID: 15310150.

Walker, Amy H., Derek Najarian, David L. White, Julie M. Jaffe, Peter A. Kanetsky, and Timothy R. Rebbeck, "Collection of Genomic DNA by Buccal Swabs for Polymerase Chain Reaction–Based Biomarker Assays," *Environmental Health Perspectives*, Vol. 107, No. 7, July 1999, pp. 517–520, PMID: 10378997.

Wang, Sophia S., Mark E. Sherman, Janet S. Rader, Joseph Carreon, Mark Schiffman, and Carl C. Baker, "Cervical Tissue Collection Methods for RNA Preservation: Comparison of Snap-Frozen, Ethanol-Fixed, and RNAlater-Fixation," *Diagnostic Molecular Pathology*, Vol. 15, No. 3, September 2006, pp. 144–148, PMID: 16932069.

Wester, Kenneth, Anna Asplund, Helena Bäckvall, Patrick Micke, Andra Derveniece, Ilona Hartmane, Per-Uno Malmström, and Fredrik Pontén, "Zinc-Based Fixative Improves Preservation of Genomic DNA and Proteins in Histoprocessing of Human Tissues," *Laboratory Investigation*, Vol. 83, No. 6, June 2003, pp. 889–899, PMID: 12808124.

Williams, Cecilia, Fredrik Pontén, Catherine Moberg, Peter Söderkvist, Mathias Uhlén, Jan Pontén, Gisela Sitbon, and Joakim Lundeberg, "A

High Frequency of Sequence Alterations Is Due to Formalin Fixation of Archival Specimens," *American Journal of Pathology*, Vol. 155, No. 5, November 1999, pp. 1467–1471, PMID: 10550302.

Yang, Wen, Botoul Maqsodi, Yunqing Ma, Son Bui, Kimberly L. Crawford, Gary K. McMaster, Frank Witney, and Yuling Luo, "Direct Quantification of Gene Expression in Homogenates of Formalin-Fixed, Paraffin-Embedded Tissues," *BioTechniques*, Vol. 40, No. 4, April 2006, pp. 481–486; erratum in *BioTechniques*, Vol. 40, No. 5, May 2006, p. 596, PMID: 16629395.

Zsikla, V., M. Baumann, and G. Cathomas, "Effect of Buffered Formalin on Amplification of DNA from Paraffin Wax Embedded Small Biopsies Using Real-Time PCR," *Journal of Clinical Pathology*, Vol. 57, No. 6, June 2004, pp. 654–656, PMID: 15166276.

REFERENCES

Barker, Anna D., Carolyn C. Compton, Julie Schneider, Jim Vaught, and Rihab Yasin, "Harmonizing Processes and Policies for NCI-Supported Biorepositories," presentation to National Cancer Advisory Board, September 20, 2005.

Eastmond, Dawn L., and Hillary C. M. Nelson, "Genome-Wide Analysis Reveals New Roles for the Activation Domains of the *Saccharomyces cerevisiae* Heat Shock Transcription Factor (Hsf1) During the Transient Heat Shock Response," *Journal of Biological Chemistry*, Vol. 281, No. 43, October 2006, pp. 32909–32921.

Eiseman, Elisa, Gabrielle Bloom, Jennifer Brower, Noreen Clancy, and Stuart S. Olmsted, *Case Studies of Existing Human Tissue Repositories: "Best Practices" for a Biospecimen Resource for the Genomic and Proteomic Era*, Santa Monica, Calif.: RAND Corporation, MG-120-NDC/NCI, 2003. As of May 5, 2009: http://www.rand.org/pubs/monographs/MG120/

Eiseman, Elisa, and Joseph B. Bolen, "Engagement of the High-Affinity IgE Receptor Activates src Protein-Related Tyrosine Kinases," *Nature*, Vol. 355, January 2, 1992, pp. 78–80.

Eiseman, Elisa, and Susanne B. Haga, *Handbook of Human Tissue Sources: A National Resource of Human Tissue Samples*, Santa Monica, Calif.: RAND Corporation, MR-954-OSTP, 1999. As of May 5, 2009: http://www.rand.org/pubs/monograph_reports/MR954/

Kawasaki, Shinji, Chris Borchert, Michael Deyholos, Hong Wang, Susan Brazille, Kiyoshi Kawai, David Galbraith, and Hans J. Bohnert, "Gene Expression Profiles During the Initial Phase of Salt Stress in Rice," *Plant Cell*, Vol. 13, No. 4, April 2001, pp. 889–906.

Kenneth, Niall Steven, and Sonia Rocha, "Regulation of Gene Expression by Hypoxia," *Biochemical Journal*, Vol. 414, 2008, pp. 19–29.

National Cancer Institute Office of Biorepositories and Biospecimen Research, homepage, undated (a). As of May 14, 2009: http://biospecimens.cancer.gov/

———, "About OBBR: Historical Milestones," Web page, undated (b). As of May 14, 2009: http://biospecimens.cancer.gov/about/

———, "About OBBR: Overview," Web page, undated (c). As of May 12, 2009: http://biospecimens.cancer.gov/about/overview.asp

———, "Welcome to the Biospecimen Research Database," Web page, undated (d). As of May 14, 2009: https://brd.nci.nih.gov/BRN/brnHome.seam

National Center for Biotechnology Information, "MeSH," Web page, undated. As of May 14, 2009: http://www.ncbi.nlm.nih.gov/sites/entrez?db=mesh

National Library of Medicine, "Fact Sheet: Medical Subject Headings (MeSH®)," last updated December 15, 2008. As of May 14, 2009: http://www.nlm.nih.gov/pubs/factsheets/mesh.html

NCBI—*see* National Center for Biotechnology Information.

NLM—*see* National Library of Medicine.

OBBR—*see* National Cancer Institute Office of Biorepositories and Biospecimen Research.

Steinberg, Christian E. W., Stephen R. Stürzenbaum, and Ralph Menzel, "Genes and Environment: Striking the Fine Balance Between Sophisticated Biomonitoring and True Functional Environmental Genomics," *Science of the Total Environment*, Vol. 400, Nos. 1–3, August 1, 2008, pp. 142–161.

Storey, K. B., and J. M. Storey, eds., *Environmental Stressors and Gene Responses*, Vol. 1: *Cell and Molecular Responses to Stress*, Amsterdam: Elsevier, 2000.

Van Elzen, Roos, Luc Moens, and Sylvia Dewilde, "Expression Profiling of the Cerebral Ischemic and Hypoxic Response," *Expert Review of Proteomics*, Vol. 5, No. 2, 2008, pp. 263–282.